BREAKING FREE WORKBOOK

Overcoming Common Problems Series

A full list of titles is available from
Sheldon Press, 36 Causton Street, London SW1P 4ST
and on our website at www.sheldonpress.co.uk

Overcoming Common Problems Series

Overcoming Common Problems Series

BREAKING FREE WORKBOOK

Carolyn Ainscough
and Kay Toon

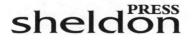

Published in Great Britain in 2000

Society for Promoting Christian Knowledge
36 Causton Street
London SW1P 4ST

British Library Cataloguing-in-Publication Data
A catalogue record for this book is available from the British Library

ISBN 978–0–85969–804–7

Typeset by Wilmaset Ltd, Birkenhead, Wirral
First printed in Great Britain by Whitstable Litho, Whitstable, Kent
Reprinted in Great Britain by Ashford Colour Press

Produced on paper from sustainable forests

Contents

Preface

Breaking Free Workbook is for male and female Survivors of childhood sexual abuse and guides you step by step through a series of exercises aimed at recognizing, understanding and working on the problems resulting from childhood abuse. The workbook is a companion book to *Breaking Free: Help for Survivors of Child Sexual Abuse* (1993, new edition 2000).

Since *Breaking Free* was first published we have continued to work with Survivors of sexual abuse referred to the Adult Psychological Therapies Service of Wakefield and Pontefract Community (NHS) Trust. We also work outside the health service providing training and consultancy to people around the country who work with Survivors of childhood sexual abuse. We have received feedback from many Survivors describing how *Breaking Free* has helped them understand more about sexual abuse and encouraged them to work on their problems by themselves or with professional support. Therapists have also told us that they found the book useful when working with Survivors. Many people have told us they would like something more. They wanted to know more on a practical level about how to overcome the problems resulting from sexual abuse and about the difficulties that are often encountered. The workbook has been written as a practical guide primarily for Survivors. We also hope therapists will find these exercises useful for working with Survivors individually or in groups. Many Survivors have contributed their own completed exercises to this book and have also written about their experiences of doing the exercises. We hope this helps to give a fuller picture of the process of healing – the struggles and the setbacks as well as what helps Survivors cope and move on.

Although there has been an increase in public awareness of child abuse in recent years there is still much to be done to prevent child abuse and to help adult Survivors who are still suffering. We hope this workbook will help contribute to Survivors taking control of their lives, feeling more confident and fulfilling their potential. We continue to believe in the powerful effects of breaking the silence about child abuse and to feel inspired by Survivors' strength to heal and to grow.

Acknowledgements

The exercises in this book developed over a number of years from our work with Survivors from Wakefield and Pontefract and we would like to thank all those Survivors for sharing their experiences and for inspiring us with their courage. We particularly want to thank the Survivors who over the last year completed draft exercises, gave suggestions and comments and generously contributed their writings to this book. We would also like to thank Survivors from the support network Moving On for their many contributions and for their constant enthusiasm and encouragement. Thanks to Leslie Cohen, Jon Fraise and Sue Richardson for their comments on the Introduction and to Mary Penford for providing illustrations for the Chapter on Mothers.

Carolyn Ainscough and Kay Toon

Many friends have helped during the writing of this book and I would like to thank the following people for giving their time and supporting me by reading through the many drafts of the book, for feeding back helpful suggestions and for their encouragement: Chris Bethlehem, Em Edmondson, Diane Skinner and James Taylor. Writing a book inevitably takes time away from families and friends and I would like especially to thank Jerry Hardman-Jones, Kirstie, Catriona, John and Tag, for their patience and support throughout the development of this book.

Kay Toon

My thanks to Margaret Ainscough, Andrew Lister and Mandy McFarlane for reading through draft chapters and for their thoughtful comments.

Carolyn Ainscough

Introduction

> I have walked through the valley of the shadow of death and emerged into sunlight, stronger. I am no longer an empty shell. I look forward to living everyday. There is joy in the simple things of life. Fear no longer grips me. I feel that I am able to breathe and that I have a right to live. CALLI

There are millions of Survivors of childhood sexual abuse in Britain alone and now more and more are speaking out and finding ways to break free from their past. In our last book *Breaking Free: Help for Survivors of Sexual Abuse* (1993, new edition 2000) many Survivors from Wakefield spoke out about what had happened to them. We know that their courage has helped other Survivors to face their own past and to take the first steps towards a better future. *Breaking Free Workbook* draws on the background information in *Breaking Free* and focuses on practical exercises to work step-by-step on problems that result from being sexually abused as a child. It is a companion book to *Breaking Free* and the two books can be used separately or together. Many Survivors have completed these exercises and contributed their writings and experiences to this book. The exercises are designed to help you think in a new way about your past, gradually break free from the problems that are disrupting your life and look forward to your future.

Is this book for me?

This book is for male and female Survivors of childhood sexual abuse who want to explore the effects of their experiences and work on their current difficulties. Sexual abuse is any kind of sexual behaviour by an adult with a child, or any unwanted or inappropriate sexual behaviour from another child. Your abuser may have been a man or a woman; you may have been abused by one person, many different individuals or you may have been abused by a group of people. You will find more information about what sexual abuse is and the terms we use in this book at the end of this chapter.

Being sexually abused as a child affects people to differing degrees. How you have been affected will depend on a number of factors including who abused you; how long the abuse went on for; how old you were when it started and ended (or it may still be ongoing); what was done and said to you; and if you had any good experiences, support, or care in your childhood. Some Survivors will be able to come to terms with what has happened to them by themselves, by seeking support and help from family and friends, or by using this self-help book. Some Survivors may also need to seek professional help from a therapist or mental health worker. Every Survivor's experience is unique and each Survivor will need different levels of help and support.

The exercises in this book can be painful at times but they can also be very beneficial. However, they need to be used with caution as they can bring up strong feelings and have powerful effects. Your safety and well-being are of the utmost importance and you need to think about what level of support you require.

- You can use this book on your own but we recommend that you think about sources of support before you start (see Chapter 1).
- If you are already receiving counselling, psychological or psychiatric help or taking medication for psychological problems we advise you to speak to your therapist or doctor before embarking on these exercises. Your therapist or counsellor may be happy to work through this book with you.
- If you have severe problems or engage in life-threatening behaviour, such as serious self-harm, only use this book with the help of a professional mental health worker.

We know that many Survivors can be helped by these exercises but we do not pretend to have any magical answers to your problems. It *is* possible to break free from the damaging effects of sexual abuse but this can take time. You may have had problems over many years and they won't just disappear overnight. This book is not intended as a substitute for professional help – in fact we hope that completing this workbook might encourage some of you to seek further help. Many of the exercises in this book are also useful for people who have been physically or emotionally abused as children.

About this book

This book focuses on practical ways to identify and change harmful beliefs and behaviours resulting from being sexually abused as a child. It also aims to help you work through your feelings about the abuse and feel better about yourself. In each chapter there are exercises for you to do, and charts and checklists to fill in. The exercises are in a step-by-step format with each exercise building on what was done in the previous exercise. There is space in the book to complete the exercises so you can build up your own record of your journey towards healing. There are examples of the exercises completed by both male and female Survivors. Survivors have also commented on the benefits and difficulties of these exercises and what helped them cope.

Part I Beginnings: Understanding your Present Problems and Keeping Safe

Chapter 1 looks at how to keep safe whilst using this book. It is important to read this chapter first as it will help you prepare for difficulties that might arise by looking at sources of support and how to look after yourself whilst doing the exercises. Chapter 2 begins the process of helping you face your own past experiences and linking them to present problems. Chapter 3 helps you to become aware of the coping strategies that you currently use and to move to consciously using non-harmful coping strategies. Chapter 4 helps you identify and deal with the things that trigger extreme feelings and behaviours, flashbacks and hallucinations.

Part II Guilt and Self Blame

Chapters 5, 6 and 7 are about the feelings of guilt and self-blame that Survivors so often experience. Many Survivors believe they are responsible for being abused because they didn't stop the abuse or didn't tell anyone, or because they think they caused the abuse to happen. The exercises in the chapters help you to challenge these kind of beliefs and to understand that the responsibility for abuse always lies with the abuser and never with the abused child.

Part III Feelings about Yourself and Others

Chapter 8 (Abusers) is about exploring your feelings towards your abuser(s) and regaining your own power. Chapter 9 (Mothers) contains exercises to help you explore your feelings about your mother (or any other person who didn't sexually abuse you as a child and should have protected you). Chapter 10 (Childhood) helps you to look back on yourself as a child, and to communicate with and nurture the child you were. It also helps you understand why you might have difficulties relating to children.

Part IV Looking to the Future

Chapter 11 helps you to assess the progress you have made so far and to look at what further steps you might want to take in the future.

This book is a first step towards healing, rather than a final solution. We hope it will give you the confidence to break free of your past by sharing your experiences with others, contacting other Survivors of sexual abuse and going for professional help. The resources section at the end of the book gives details about where you can seek further help.

Is this the right time to use this workbook?

When is the right time to work on your abuse? Many Survivors are frightened about the consequences of working on their abuse. This is understandable. Doing anything different is a risk. If you have coped in the past by trying to forget about your abuse, doing these exercises is a radically different approach and it will take a leap of faith to get started. The exercise below will help you examine what is standing in your way and to decide if this is the right time to start this workbook.

EXERCISE 1   IS THIS THE RIGHT TIME?

Aim   To help you think about whether this is the right time to start using this workbook and to understand more about what might be stopping you looking at the abuse and working on your difficulties.

Below are a number of reasons given by Survivors for not starting to work on their past abuse and current difficulties. Tick off any of the reasons that apply to you and add any others you can think of below.

Current situation:	Applies to you?
Examinations	
Relationship break up	
Pregnant	
Just started a new job	
Just started a new relationship	

Fear of:	
What you might feel	
What you might remember	
Not being able to cope	
What your family/partner/friends will think	
The consequences of beginning to change	
Being hurt or rejected	

When you are feeling depressed or anxious saying to yourself:

I'm depressed and I don't want to make things worse	
I'm depressed and I don't have the resources to cope	

When you are feeling OK saying to yourself:

I'm OK and I don't want to risk making myself depressed again	
I'm OK and everything is sorted out now	

Thinking (or being told):	Applies to you?
You should look forward rather than dwelling on the past	_____
You are making a mountain out of a mole hill	_____
Your experiences and problems are too great to be sorted out	_____
Your problems will go away by themselves	_____
Too busy – putting other things or other people first	_____
Being unsure whether your memories are of real events	_____
_____	_____
_____	_____
_____	_____
_____	_____
_____	_____
_____	_____
_____	_____

Survivor's comment

The exercises need to be carried out when you are ready to face issues otherwise there is minimal progress. It is about daring to believe the truth and step-by-step becoming stronger in that belief. CATH

Current situation

If you are in a particular crisis at the moment or have something very important that you have to deal with right now, you may wish to wait until you feel more stable or have more space and time to cope with doing this work.

I think the right time to do these exercises is when you are out of the abusive situation with a safe place to live and you become aware that there is a recurrent problem that you want to try to solve. CATHERINE

I think it could be the wrong time to do the exercises if you are feeling extremely stressed or uncomfortable. It may mean you have to do them in small portions but at least you will be doing them from a position of strength which is always best. REBECCA

Everyone is individual but I think you need to be ready to do the exercises. I think it is difficult if your present-day situation is in turmoil, e.g. marriage break-up, loss and grief or if you have no outside support. SARAH

If you do not feel ready to work on the exercises at the moment you may feel able to read *Breaking Free* now and return to this workbook later.

It might be painful

Many people try to cope with sexual abuse by blocking off their memories and feelings. This is one of the few ways in which children are able to cope but this strategy has disadvantages. It doesn't work completely and it doesn't last. Bad feelings and memories 'escape' as nightmares, panic attacks, fears, depression, sexual difficulties, flashbacks and many other problems. These problems are the symptoms of the underlying trauma of being sexually abused. It can be difficult to get rid of the symptoms until the underlying problem is dealt with.

Working on your past experiences and current problems is not an easy task. It will probably bring up feelings and memories that are painful and hard to cope with. However, you would probably not be reading this book if you were totally happy with the way things are for you at the moment. Working on yourself can be hard but it is also very rewarding. Many Survivors feel that by working on themselves they become more aware of who they are and what they want and begin to see a way through their problems.

I'm OK/I'm depressed

Many Survivors alternate between feeling reasonably OK and then having bouts of depression or anxiety or even feeling suicidal. When you are feeling OK, understandably you want to believe that all your problems have gone away and will not come back. Although people can often block out their feelings and memories for a time and feel OK, they cannot do this all the time and then they experience another period of depression or anxiety. Look back over the last few years of your life and see if you recognize this pattern. Working on your abuse will mean facing painful feelings but it can also help you break free from this pattern of plunging in and out of periods of extreme emotions.

It's in the past

Survivors are often told 'it's in the past, forget about it'. Friends and family who hear you talking about the abuse or see your distress may often feel uncomfortable and not know what to do or how to respond. Saying 'forget about it' might be a way of refusing to get involved or might be a genuine attempt to be helpful. It isn't. Unfortunately doctors and health workers also sometimes give this unhelpful advice. You may have also said this to yourself. If you could forget about the past and not be affected by it you would. No one wants to dwell on unhappy events or create problems just for the sake of it. Past events need to be brought into full awareness, understood and processed before we can truly let go of them and move on.

If you remember and relive the hurt and pain you went through it will help you to put it to the back of your mind and start to live a normal life. I thought the idea was to try to forget but I realize now that I will never forget what they did to me. I'm not after forgetting, I'm after trying to understand and to come to terms with it. JEAN

I'm making a mountain out of a mole hill

The sexual abuse of a child is a serious crime and a trauma that should not have to be endured. It is normal to experience difficulties when you have been traumatized. Trying to face your difficulties and deal with them is a courageous act. It isn't moaning and making a fuss about nothing.

What will other people think?

You cannot control what other people will think and feel about your decision to work on your abuse. Some people will be supportive but others may be hostile. Sometimes people do not understand about the effects of abuse and may think that you are getting worse if you are crying or getting angry. They may want to try and stop you continuing with these exercises because they are trying to protect you or because they feel it would be easier for them if you remained silent about what has happened. It is normal to feel angry and upset about being abused and you have a right to express your feelings and speak about what has happened to you if you want to. During the abuse your feelings were ignored and you had to remain silent. Now you have a chance to begin to undo the wrongs that have been done to you.

Did it really happen?

Sometimes Survivors wonder whether the abuse really happened or whether they are imagining it. This can be more of a problem if:

- You do not have complete memories.
- You blocked memories of the abuse for a period of time and have now got access to them again.
- Your memories and feelings are surfacing in flashbacks and dreams.
- You were in a confused state of mind during the abuse because you were half asleep or intoxicated with alcohol or drugs or did not really understand what was happening.
- Your abuser has denied the abuse.
- Your abuser was also warm and caring.
- Other people have not believed you.
- You have read about people having so-called 'False Memory Syndrome'.
- You coped with the abuse as a child by pretending it was a dream or that it was happening to someone else.
- What you remember seems too extreme or bizarre to be true.

Many Survivors have these worries and difficulties. Pretending the abuse didn't happen and blocking out painful memories and feelings is a very common way of coping with any kind of trauma and can leave people feeling very confused about what has really happened. Some Survivors say that they have lost access to all memories of their abuse for periods of time even when there is concrete evidence about what has happened to them. Memories of the past can be triggered by current events such as the birth of a baby or the death of an abuser. Memories of frightening events may also be accessed again when you begin to feel safe or strong enough to deal with them. If you do not have full memories you may be anxious to find out what happened to you; however, this is not something that can be forced. Survivors often get access to memories gradually and this helps to protect them from becoming overwhelmed. Memories can also become distorted over time and some Survivors may never know for sure exactly what happened to them. However, you do not need to have full and exact memories to use this workbook. Doing these exercises can help you explore your feelings and beliefs and develop a new understanding of yourself and your experiences.

Some people have no memories of abuse but suffer from various symptoms and problems that make them wonder whether they have been abused. It is not possible to 'diagnose' a past history of sexual abuse from current problems and symptoms and this book cannot tell you whether or not you have been sexually abused. If you have no memories of abuse but have symptoms and difficulties you wish to deal with it is advisable to consult a therapist rather than using this book.

Writing

All the chapters contain exercises which ask you to write about your feelings and experiences. Many Survivors find that writing plays a very important part in their recovery. Some Survivors find the idea of writing very threatening and may also feel that it won't be helpful. Writing can make the reality of what has happened very clear and although this can be frightening it can also be very healing.

> Writing made me face up to the reality of the abuse. It helped me acknowledge the abuse instead of trying to shut it away. I could no longer deny it. I was frightened but it does get better. It was worth it in the end. MAYA

Writing isn't the same as just thinking things out. Many Survivors recall memories and feelings and begin to understand themselves better once they begin to write.

You may feel anxious about writing and feel you will fail or make a mess of things. The education of many Survivors has suffered because of abuse during childhood. You may have been punished or laughed at or called stupid. Try to remember that this is not a test of your writing. The writing is for you to get access to your thoughts and feelings, so spelling, grammar and style don't matter.

There are many ways of writing your answers to the exercises. You don't need to write in the style of an essay. You could write a list or write down key words. You could make out a chart or a diagram. Many Survivors enjoy writing poetry – you could answer the exercises in poems. Do whatever feels easiest and most comfortable for you. If you have trouble writing you could speak into a tape recorder, get someone you trust to write as you speak or use one of the alternatives to writing described below.

The writing is for your benefit. It is not necessary for anyone else to read it. If you are worried that someone else might find your writing, keep it in a safe place or leave it in a sealed envelope with someone you trust. Writing can also be a good way of communicating your experiences and feelings to other people without having to talk, so you may *want* to share your writing with someone else. Sharing your writing also helps to break the secrecy of your abuse.

Survivors' comments

Keep a daily diary of what you do in your life – even little things, especially if they are positive. This will:

- Provide you with an outline of your experiences.
- Show your progress.
- Remind you of how brave you have been.
- Remind you of positive and happy things that have happened to you.
- Be a record of a very important part of your life and development as a person.

It is important to write the date on all your writings and keep them somewhere safe. I find this really helps me see how I am progressing and pulls experiences together that might otherwise be forgotten. Also record your dreams – they can be very significant in suggesting you are making progress on a deeper level. ANNABELLE

I was so programmed into a 'don't tell or else' dogma that I thought I would suffer a fate worse than death if I wrote things down. Luckily I had a very supportive counsellor who let me work on the writing during our sessions and helped allay my fears. I took it step-by-step until I gained confidence and became angry about the abuse. I have found my own personal power now and it is a good feeling to know that I can write and that this is a valuable resource. As you can see I am not frightened of writing anymore. MAYA

The exercises have got me to write which I've always avoided. Before, when I thought about the past I pushed it to one side. Now I think I haven't got to bury it deep in my head. I'm writing it down and finding it helpful. It's one way of getting it out of my system although it hurts. I never wanted to read in black and white what my abuser did but now I'm beginning to realize that the only way I can do something about my problems is by recognizing what he did and fighting back. By writing it down you can break the hold he has on you. I feel now I want to write and write and write. The more I write the easier it is getting. I feel like I am never going to stop. There is so much to write and get out of my system. JEAN

Alternatives to writing

Not everyone feels comfortable with writing. In some of the exercises in the book we have suggested alternatives to writing. You could also try to adapt the other exercises and use one of the methods below.

Drawing, painting, using art materials

When you are asked to write about an event or about how you feel, you may feel happier drawing, painting or using art materials in other ways. You could draw stick figures or a sequence of events like a cartoon. You could also use clay or Plasticine to sculpt objects or scenes. Some Survivors have made collages to represent their answers to the exercises. Painting can be a powerful way of expressing your feelings and colour can be used to represent different feelings, different people or different times of your life. You do not have to be artistic in any way to use these methods. The aim is not to create a work of art but to find a different way of expressing your thoughts and feelings and getting in touch with ideas and feelings you may not be consciously aware of.

Talking

If you find talking easier than writing you could talk through the exercises with another person or use the technique of **talking to an empty chair**. Sit in a chair with an empty chair opposite you and imagine that another person is sitting on that chair. This 'other person' could be someone you know and trust, an imaginary safe person or a part of yourself. Talk through the exercises with this person. Talk out loud rather than in your head. You could try talking through the exercises as a first step towards writing.

The words we use

Sexual abuse

We use the term 'sexual abuse' to mean any kind of sexual behaviour by an adult with a child or any unwanted or inappropriate sexual behaviour from another child. This includes sexual intercourse, oral sex, anal sex, being touched in a sexual way and being persuaded to touch someone else. It may involve inserting objects into the child's body or sexual acts with animals. However, sexual abuse doesn't always involve physical contact. Being made to watch other people's sexual behaviour, or to look at their bodies or at sexual photographs or videos can also be forms of sexual abuse. Sexual abuse includes abuse by one person, abuse by a number of different people or by groups of people. The abuse may have happened only once or many times over a number of years. It may still be happening now.

Abusers

An abuser is anyone who has sexually abused a child. This could be a father, mother, brother, other family member, friend, person in authority, acquaintance, older child or a stranger. Although the majority of abusers are thought to be men (maybe 80 per cent) many Survivors have been abused by women.

Child

The word 'child' is used here to refer to teenagers as well as younger children. Abuse can start as a teenager or in adulthood. This book is primarily for people whose sexual abuse started before they became adults.

Survivors

We use the word 'Survivors' to refer to men and women who have been sexually abused as children. They have had to find ways of surviving the trauma of sexual abuse but, with the help of this book, we hope they will go beyond simply surviving to living a fuller and happier life.

Survivors and abusers can come from any walk of life or any religious or ethnic background.

Many Survivors have contributed their writings to this book to share with you their struggles, their experiences, their hopes and their successes.

> The chaos in my head was too big to handle on my own. I needed help to break it down so I could work it out. To try to think things through yourself is daunting. The exercises managed to organize my thoughts into smaller parts so I could consider them more thoroughly. I also need prompting before I think about my abuse – the exercises provided that prompt. I am now more positive and able to communicate. The exercises have helped me to feel more self-confident and in control of my life. CATHERINE

This book does not contain all the answers to your problems but it could be a first step towards breaking free of your past and beginning to move on. Now make sure you turn to the next chapter which gives advice on how to use the workbook and how to keep safe whilst doing the exercises. Good luck with the work ahead.

I

Beginnings:
Understanding Your
Present Problems
and Keeping Safe

This section helps you to understand more about how the abuse has affected your life and about ways of coping and keeping safe. Chapter 2 helps you focus on your present problems and explains how sexual abuse can lead to problems. Chapters 1, 3 and 4 look at how to keep safe and how to deal with difficult feelings, memories and symptoms.

1
How to Use this Book and Keep Safe

This chapter contains suggestions about how to do the exercises in this book and helps you find ways of keeping safe whilst doing them. The exercises are designed to help you challenge your beliefs, reassess your past and process your feelings. Working on your thoughts and feelings about the past can be very distressing so it is important that you have some control over how deeply you get into your feelings. As a child you were treated as though your feelings did not matter. The sexual abuse was to satisfy the desires of the abuser; how you felt was not important to him or her. You are important and it does matter how you feel. It is important that you take care of yourself whilst you do these exercises, that you move through them at your own pace and that you feel in control of what you are going through. This chapter looks at what you need to know before you start the exercises, how to protect yourself and create the right emotional distance whilst you are doing the exercises, and how to look after yourself when you have completed an exercise. Work carefully through this section and spend some time ensuring you know how to keep yourself safe before you begin the exercises in the rest of this book.

Before you start the exercises

Where to start

- We recommend that you do the exercises in the order they appear in the book. The chapters build on each other and follow the sequence we have found to be most helpful for Survivors of sexual abuse. Sometimes you may want to go back and do some of the exercises again or occasionally you may need to jump ahead, for example to look at how to deal with a disturbing symptom such as a flashback.
- Some exercises may seem too frightening or too difficult. Don't force yourself to do exercises you don't feel ready for. You may be able to return to them later

when you feel stronger or have more support. All the exercises may not be suitable or necessary for everyone.

- The exercises in Chapters 3 and 4 help you to understand more about the kind of difficult experiences and reactions that Survivors commonly have. Working through these chapters before moving on to the rest of the book will help you keep safe and feel more in control of what is happening to you.
- Many of the exercises are followed by examples and comments from Survivors. You might want to look through these before you begin an exercise.
- You can photocopy the exercises in this book. If you have more than one abuser you will need to repeat some of the exercises for each of your abusers.
- Refer back to this chapter before, during or after each exercise if you need to remind yourself of ways to keep safe and take care of yourself.

Getting support

It may sometimes be hard to cope alone whilst you are working through this book. If you are feeling depressed you may feel very alone and think that no one understands or wants to help. Often there are people around – friends, family, local services and organizations – who would be willing to help. When you are feeling really bad it can be difficult to find out about services or to ask for help for the first time so try to do this preparation work now. At the back of the book is a list of organizations who could provide help. The national organizations listed will often be able to give information about local contacts. You could also ask your community health council or social services about what resources are available in your local area. Getting help and support from others is a useful and practical way of dealing with your problems, *not* a sign of weakness and failure. You might want to ask a friend to act as a support person while you work through this book. If you do start to feel overwhelmed and cannot cope, seek professional help – your GP will be able to advise you.

EXERCISE 1.1   SOURCES OF HELP

Aim   To find sources of help for yourself and to have a ready-made list of contacts to refer to when you are feeling bad.

Make a list of people you could telephone when you are feeling bad. You may want to include national and local helplines such as the Samaritans, friends, family members, and professional workers who may be involved with your care. Your GP should be contacted in case of emergencies or if you are feeling suicidal; add his/her number to your list.

Name	Telephone number	Times available

Also make a list of people or organizations you could visit or ask to visit you.

Name	Address/telephone number	Times available

Survivor's comment

I think you have to be ready in your own mind for anything the exercises bring up and ask for help if you need it. LESLEY-LEIGH

Making preparations

You will need to take time to do these exercises and prepare yourself for any strong emotional reactions. Set aside time to work through this book and do the exercises in a place where you feel safe and comfortable. For some of you this may be somewhere where you are alone and undisturbed, others may want to have people around. You may want to think about how much time you are going to devote to these exercises at one sitting. You will need to give yourself plenty of time to work on the exercise and to deal with your reactions afterwards. Do not expect to do too much at one go. These exercises can bring up powerful feelings and can be very tiring. You may want to have a support person with you when you do the exercises or available afterwards. Some Survivors find comfort by having a special object, such as a soft toy, with them whilst doing the exercises. Think about what would feel best for you and make some notes below.

Place _____

Time of day _____

How much time to spend at one go? _____

Who would you like with you? _____

Who would you like available afterwards? _____

What special object would you like with you? _____

Survivors' comments

> I found I was reluctant to start the exercises. I was tense and panicky and aware that my husband was around. I overcame my difficulties in starting by asking my husband to go out (and I told him why!). I was then able to concentrate on the exercise. MAYA

> I did not want to do the exercises when I was alone or late at night. REBECCA

During the exercises

This book aims to help you understand and process your memories and feelings. This is not easy to do if you become flooded by your memories and overwhelmed by your feelings. You therefore need to set a pace that is comfortable for you and to approach the exercises from a safe emotional distance.

Going at your own pace

There is no right speed at which you should progress through this work book. Some people will work through the book quickly, others will complete the exercises slowly, maybe leaving gaps of time before moving on to the next section. It is up to you to set the pace that feels comfortable for you.

When should I slow down? It is advisable to slow down if you find yourself being overwhelmed by feelings, behaving in harmful ways or unable to process your thoughts and feelings. You may wish to take a break from the exercises for a while. Some Survivors come back to the same exercises again and again before they feel they are ready to move on. If you begin to experience strong emotional or physical reactions allow yourself time and space to understand and process these reactions before continuing with the next exercises.

When should I speed up? You need to work at your own pace rather than pushing yourself to work faster because you think you ought to. If you know other people who are using this workbook try not to compare yourself with them. Everyone is unique in their reactions and needs. However, if you are picking this workbook up, doing a little and then forgetting about it for weeks and months, it may be helpful to look at why you might be avoiding doing this work and what reasons you are giving yourself for this. Look back at Exercise 1, on page xii.

Survivors' comments

> It helped me contain my feelings by working through the exercises in bits although I was always tempted to move straight on to the next chapter. I also

made sure I was in a safe place where I could contact people if I needed to. THOMAS

I found some of the exercises too powerful to do in one go so I spaced them out over a couple of hours with some fun things in between. REBECCA

Finding a safe distance

Learn how to feel safe before attempting the exercises. REBECCA

To do the exercises in this book you will need to think about your past and get in touch with your feelings. If you have pushed your memories and feelings away or if you cut off and feel numb while you are doing the exercises it may be helpful to get closer to your experiences in order to work on them. On the other hand, if you are constantly overwhelmed by your memories and feelings then you may not be able to do the thinking required by these exercises or process what is happening to you. If you are either too close to or too far from your feelings and experiences, it can be difficult to benefit from these exercises. Below are a number of ways in which you can try to create the emotional distance that feels safe for you whilst doing these exercises.

Creating distance from your experiences

Feeling overwhelmed by your feelings is distressing and can make it difficult for you to do the exercises. It is therefore helpful to know how to distance yourself from your memories and feelings whilst doing these exercises. Pushing your experiences away and distracting yourself in the short term can be very useful ways of protecting yourself and giving yourself a break from feeling bad. As you feel stronger you may be able to repeat the exercises from a closer position. Below is a list of ways of containing painful feelings, creating distance and doing the exercises in a cooler way.

You can cope with overwhelming memories and feelings by:

- Trying to become aware of how you usually push your thoughts and feelings away or distract yourself, and then using these techniques consciously.
- Stopping in the middle of an exercise if necessary and using a coping strategy (see Chapter 3).

Survivors have suggested the following techniques to symbolically rid yourself of bad feelings and contain painful memories for a while.

- Put your bad feelings on a rug or blanket and shake it out of the door.
- Run water over your wrists to wash your feelings away.
- Put your memories in a box and lock it.

Below are distancing techniques that can be used with exercises which ask you to write about yourself or think about an incident or person or look at photographs.

- Imagine you are writing about someone else rather than yourself and write in the third person, e.g. 'Mandy (rather than 'I') has problems with eating; she often binge-eats when she is upset.'
- Choose an incident that is not too distressing for you or at a level of distress you can cope with. There is no need to dive into the worst incidents first.
- If you have several abusers, work on the abuser you feel least frightened of or disturbed by first.
- If it feels too painful to think about yourself as a child think about another child (a child you know or an imaginary child) rather than yourself.
- Look at incidents or people as if through the wrong end of a telescope or binoculars so they appear smaller and further away and have a less powerful effect.
- Imagine you are watching the person (it may be you) or incident on a video and you have the remote control. You can stop it or pause it so you are in control of how much you see and hear.

Survivors' comments

Use your own way of pushing away your memories or feelings to a safe distance. Persevere. Even if you are frightened like I was during the exercises it does get better. It's worth it in the end. Say positive affirmations to yourself like 'I can do this and I will'. MAYA

When I feel really bad I breathe in deeply then blow my breath out through pursed lips and try to blow all my bad feelings out into the air with my breath. I sometimes move my arms about to help push the bad feelings away. ALMA

Getting closer to the experience

Use the techniques below only if you think you are too cut off from your feelings or out of touch with your experiences.

- Look at photographs of yourself as a child, your abuser, your family or where you used to live.
- Spend some time sitting quietly and try to become aware of what you are feeling. Focus on any body symptoms, e.g. tense shoulders, and try to stay with the feeling and become aware of what is happening within you.
- Think about a specific incident or person from your past that relates to the exercise and again try to become aware of what you are feeling.
- Hold or look at a toy or a possession you had as a child.

Remember that pushing things away can also be a way of protecting yourself from overwhelming feelings so stay in control and move only as close as you want to.

Taking care of yourself after each exercise

Take some time to look after yourself after each exercise. You may need to rest, talk to someone, get some support or find some other way of coping and taking care of yourself. Chapter 3 helps you move to using non-harmful coping strategies. If you can't finish an exercise or don't feel like you've moved on don't worry – you can try it again another time. It is normal to think a particular exercise hasn't changed anything for you. We can only change or see something in a new way when the time is right for us. Below Maya shares her experiences of coping with the after-effects of doing the exercises in this book.

- The exercise made me feel angry and I threw the paper down. I felt afraid and panicky. I played relaxing music to help me calm down. The fear increased at first – I shook from head to foot. It took time for me to realize that nothing terrible would happen to me. Now I am proud of myself for doing it and I feel stronger.
- After the exercise I felt sad that there had been no one around for me as a child so I looked after myself by climbing into my sleeping bag with my favourite cushion and playing relaxing music.
- I was extremely frightened and thought I would be found out and punished for 'lying' about the abuse. I talked to my counsellor about my fears and she supported me.
- Reward yourself after each exercise – you have taken a step towards self-understanding and personal growth. Well done! MAYA

The exercise below is about creating an imaginary safe place that you can go to whenever you feel the need to. You could go to this safe place after you have completed an exercise or whenever you feel frightened or overwhelmed.

EXERCISE 1.2 SAFE PLACE

Aim To create a safe place in your imagination that you can go to when you feel overwhelmed or unable to cope.

1 Choose a time when you are feeling reasonably OK and make yourself comfortable by lying down or sitting in a relaxed position.
2 Close your eyes and think about a place where you could be alone and feel safe, peaceful and relaxed. This could be a place that you know or a place that you imagine. Many people choose a place outside such as a deserted beach or somewhere in the countryside. If you do not feel safe being on your own, imagine that a person you feel safe with is also there.
3 Imagine that you are lying down or sitting in this place and that you are feeling warm, relaxed and safe. Concentrate on all the sensations you are experiencing. What can you see (e.g. trees, the sky, the sea)? What can you

hear (e.g. waves, birds)? What can you smell (e.g. flowers, the sea)? What can you feel (e.g. grass or sand beneath you)? Stay here for a while taking in all the sensations around you and enjoying the feeling of safety and relaxation. Remind yourself that you can come back to this place whenever you want to.

4 When you are ready open your eyes and bring yourself back to where you really are by looking round the room. Now write down a description of your safe place below and remember to include a description of what you could see, hear, smell and feel. You may want to draw or paint your safe place instead.

5 Practise going to this safe place at times when you are feeling OK until you are able to do this quite easily.

6 When you are feeling stressed, frightened, overwhelmed etc. and you need some time out, bring the image of your safe place to your mind. You can do this wherever you are; you do not need to be in a special place nor do you need to be lying down or sitting down.

MY SAFE PLACE

Examples of safe places

The air is fresh and clean, the sky clear blue. The sun shines through the trees bringing light and warmth to my garden. A stream of clear water ripples over the stones. I love to sit by the stream and listen to the sound of the water – it sings a peaceful song as it travels along. I put my cares into the stream and they are carried away. The sweet perfume of the flower garden pervades the air, reminding me of the joy of being alive. It is a special garden where the wild animals roam around freely keeping me safe from harm. The animals are my friends, they take care of me. They know when I am feeling weak – they know I will be at the stream. Gently and powerfully the lion and tiger come and rest beside me. I reach out and touch their soft fur, as I stroke them I sense their protectiveness towards me – I am safe. The water carries away my burdens and I feel free. The lion and tiger remind me that I have strength within and that I am protected. I become re-energized. As I feel the warmth of the sun on my body I can feel myself becoming alive again. CALLI

The place I imagined was on an island. It had sea all the way around. There was only one way in and that was by boat and I would see that. It had trees around with fruit on them. I had a house that I had built. I could hear the birds singing. I was protected. Every so often I would get all my friends to come and have a party. This is a nice safe place. LESLEY-LEIGH

My safe place is just after midnight on the beach at Scarborough with my wife. All the coloured lights are still lit but there are not a lot of people about. I sit on the sand which is still hot from the sun of the day. There is the sound of seagulls flying around and the purring of the beach-cleaning vehicle to make the sand clean of rubbish for the next horde of holiday-makers. Fishermen can be heard preparing their boats for the early morning trawl. A light breeze blowing every few seconds brings the smell of the cool, calm sea rippling towards us. I walk barefoot along the sand leaving footprints in the wet sand as the tide slowly starts to come in. Turning around I look back at the row of different amusement arcades lit up with hundreds of coloured bulbs. No one else is about and the whole beach is ours. The sky is black with the twinkle of stars scattered about the banana-shaped moon. Slowly the night begins to cool and the breeze brings raised pimples on our arms. This tells me that we are okay. GRAHAM

Survivors' comments

> I enjoyed going to my imaginary place and thinking about it. I have never done that before. LESLEY-LEIGH

> It's important to find a way to feel safe. I find it really hard to relax and I never feel safe. I am always watching my back and being paranoid. My husband has started to help me get through this so that I can relax a bit. My husband puts his arms around me and talks to me for a bit to reassure me that I am safe. Then I feel safe and relaxed. We are still working on this until I feel completely safe on my own. PAULA

In this chapter we have looked at ways of keeping safe and feeling more in control whilst working through this book. This is your journey and it will be challenging, but remember that whatever your feelings and reactions to the exercises you are not alone. Learning to take care of your own needs and asking for help when necessary is an important part of the healing process. We wish you well.

2
How the Abuse Has Affected My Life

When children are being sexually abused they have many confusing and distressing feelings which can also affect the way they behave. As adults many Survivors continue to have problems as a result of their childhood abuse. The problems can affect every part of their lives: how they feel, the way they think, how they relate to other people and the things they do. They may feel helpless and overwhelmed by the chaos in their lives and think it is not possible to feel better about themselves or create a better life. Many Survivors believe they have problems because they are stupid, mad, difficult, mentally ill, unsociable, bad or because they were 'born evil'. They may have been told these things by other people.

You may believe you have difficulties in your life because there is something wrong with you instead of understanding that your current problems may be a result of your past experiences. In this chapter we want to help you think more clearly about the problems you have had as an adult and understand how they might relate to your childhood abuse. You share your problems with many other Survivors, and in this book, step-by-step, we hope you will learn how to begin to overcome your problems and look forward to a brighter future.

Effects of childhood abuse

The first exercise lists the problems that are most commonly reported by Survivors of sexual abuse. However, it does not mean you have been sexually abused if you have any of these problems. This list cannot be used to 'diagnose' sexual abuse.

EXERCISE 2.1   EFFECTS OF SEXUAL ABUSE
Aim   To look at the ways that sexual abuse has affected your life and help you see that you share many of your problems with other Survivors.

Below is a list of the problems that Survivors most commonly report. Look through the list and for each problem indicate whether you currently

13

experience this problem or if you experienced it in the past. At the end of the
list add any other problems that you experience.

Problems	Applies to you?			
	Yes	*A little*	*No*	*Not now*
Fears				
Anxiety				
Phobias				
Nervousness				
Nightmares				
Sleep problems				
Depression				
Shame				
Guilt				
Feeling like a victim				
Lack of self-confidence				
Feeling different from others				
Feeling self-conscious				
Feeling unable to take action or change situations				
Feeling dirty				
Obsessed with cleaning or washing				
Constant worrying thoughts				
Suicide attempts				
Self-harming (e.g. slashing arms)				
Blackouts				
Fits				
Gaps in everyday memory				
Binge-eating				
Self-induced vomiting				
Compulsive eating				
Anorexia nervosa				
Obsessed with body image				

Problems	Applies to you?			
	Yes	*A little*	*No*	*Not now*
No interest in sex				
Fear of sex				
Avoiding specific sexual activities				
Feeling unable to say 'No' to sex				
Obsessed with sex				
Aggressive sexual behaviour				
Flashbacks (feeling of reliving parts of the past)				
Hearing the abuser's voice when he or she isn't there				
Seeing the abuser's face when he or she isn't there				
Confusion about sexual orientation (homosexual or heterosexual)				
Confusion about sexual identity (male or female)				
Unable to get close to people				
Marrying young to get away from home				
Relationship problems				
Excessive concerns about security of home or self				
Alcohol problems				
Drug problems				
Employment problems				
Being re-victimized				
Criminal involvement				

Problems	Applies to you?			
	Yes	*A little*	*No*	*Not now*
Needing to be in control	___	___	___	___
Delinquency	___	___	___	___
Aggressive behaviour	___	___	___	___
Bullying	___	___	___	___
Abusing others	___	___	___	___
Clinging and being extremely dependent	___	___	___	___
Anger	___	___	___	___
Hostility	___	___	___	___
Problems communicating	___	___	___	___
Working too hard	___	___	___	___
Distrusting people	___	___	___	___
Difficulty in being able to judge people's trustworthiness	___	___	___	___
Difficulties relating to children	___	___	___	___
Other problems				
___	___	___	___	___
___	___	___	___	___
___	___	___	___	___

Survivor's comment

Remember these are the ways you survived your abuse. Try not to be upset by all the 'Yes' responses – you can work on the underlying problems one at a time. CALLI

You may have ticked just a few of the problems on the list or many of them. You may be pleased to find you have overcome some of the difficulties you experienced in the past. It is normal to have problems as a result of traumatic experiences or inappropriate and abusive relationships. Seeing that you share your problems with other Survivors can help you realize that your problems may be a result of your abusive experiences rather than because there is something wrong with you. Being abused and unprotected as a child often results in adult Survivors having difficulties in their relationships with children, this is explored further in Chapter 10.

Many of the problems on the list above relate to things that you *do* (e.g. self-harming, avoiding sex, drinking too much); however, another important consequence of sexual abuse is the impact it has on the way you *feel*. The next two exercises explore the effects of sexual abuse on your feelings about yourself and your relationship to your emotions.

Feelings about yourself

Survivors often feel worthless because of how they were treated by their abusers and sometimes because of the lack of support or protection from other adults. The way Survivors think about the abuse also affects the way they feel about themselves. Many Survivors believe they are responsible for the abuse and this leaves them feeling guilty and ashamed. In the next exercise you are asked to think about how you feel about yourself now.

EXERCISE 2.2   FEELINGS ABOUT YOURSELF

Aim   To help you become more aware of how you feel about yourself.

Look through the following list of statements and circle the number that corresponds to how much you agree with each one. For example:

- If you totally agree with it then circle 0.
- If you neither agree nor disagree then circle 5.
- If you totally disagree then circle 10.

Feelings about myself	Agree					?				Disagree	
I hate myself	0	1	2	3	4	5	6	7	8	9	10
I don't like myself	0	1	2	3	4	5	6	7	8	9	10
I feel worthless	0	1	2	3	4	5	6	7	8	9	10
I don't accept myself	0	1	2	3	4	5	6	7	8	9	10
I am bad	0	1	2	3	4	5	6	7	8	9	10
I do not like the child I was	0	1	2	3	4	5	6	7	8	9	10
I do not feel positive about the future	0	1	2	3	4	5	6	7	8	9	10
I feel helpless	0	1	2	3	4	5	6	7	8	9	10

Your relationship to your feelings

The powerful emotions a child experiences during sexual abuse can also have long-term effects on Survivors' lives. As adults Survivors may still experience emotions such as anxiety, guilt, anger, helplessness, confusion, terror or depression. They often find it difficult to deal with these powerful feelings and may feel very uncomfortable with their own feelings. Some Survivors feel overwhelmed and frightened by their feelings whilst others cope by cutting off from their feelings and only feel 'numb'. The next exercise helps you explore your relationship with your feelings. In the last chapter you will be asked to rate your feelings again to assess any changes.

EXERCISE 2.3   YOUR RELATIONSHIP TO YOUR FEELINGS
Aim   To help you focus on how you relate to your feelings.

Look through the following list of statements and circle the number that corresponds to how much you agree with each one. For example:

- If you totally agree with it then circle 0.
- If you neither agree nor disagree then circle 5.
- If you totally disagree then circle 10.

My Feelings	Agree					?				Disagree
I am overwhelmed by my feelings	0	1	2	3	4	5	6	7	8	9	10
I am not in touch with my feelings	0	1	2	3	4	5	6	7	8	9	10
I am frightened of my own feelings	0	1	2	3	4	5	6	7	8	9	10
I am cut off from my feelings	0	1	2	3	4	5	6	7	8	9	10
I am ill at ease with my feelings	0	1	2	3	4	5	6	7	8	9	10

At this stage we are simply aiming to help you understand what problems you have and why you have them. The exercises in the rest of this book are designed to help you work through your feelings, take control of your symptoms and tackle the causes of the problems.

Survivors are affected by abuse in different ways. You are all individuals with different experiences and each of you will have found your own way of surviving the abuse. The severity of a Survivor's problems also relates to the circumstances of the abuse, such as the age of the child, the relationship with the abuser, the number of abusers, the type of abuse and the resources available to the child. A child from a caring family abused by a stranger is in a different situation and has access to more resources than a child abused by both parents with no caring adult available to him or her. Each child will be affected differently and will find his or her own way of coping.

How does sexual abuse cause these problems?

David Finkelhor, an American researcher, has tried to explain how sexual abuse affects children and leads on to the long-term problems we discussed earlier. Finkelhor suggests four processes in childhood sexual abuse which cause problems:

Traumatic Sexualization, Stigmatization, Betrayal and Powerlessness (Finkelhor, 1986). This model helps to explain how sexual abuse can fundamentally affect a person's life and is explained in more detail in *Breaking Free*.

EXERCISE 2.4   FINKELHOR'S FOUR PROCESSES
Aim   To help you understand how problems develop in Survivors' lives.

This exercise uses Finkelhor's model to help you see how sexual abuse is a traumatic experience that leads to the development of many problems in the lives of Survivors. Finkelhor's four processes are briefly described below. After each one you are asked to think about your own problems and feelings and write down which of your problems may have resulted from each process.

Traumatic sexualization
When children are sexually abused they are exposed to sexual experiences which are inappropriate or too advanced for their age or level of development. Their sexual experience, knowledge and identity are not allowed to develop naturally. They are also given confusing and incorrect messages about sexual behaviour. Their early experiences of sexual behaviour and sexuality may be traumatic. The physical and emotional pain involved in sexual abuse for many children means that sex becomes associated with bad feelings. Sometimes, however, children enjoy parts of the touching and many experience sexual pleasure and orgasm.

As a result of their inappropriate sexual experiences Survivors can grow up confused about their own sexual feelings and normal sexual behaviour. This leads to sexual difficulties in adults, ranging from fears and phobias about sex to preoccupation and obsessions with sex.

Write down any of your problems which result from traumatic sexualization:

_____
_____
_____
_____
_____
_____
_____
_____
_____
_____
_____

Examples

> When I was at school I thought everyone knew I was getting abused. I used to sleep with anybody because the abuse left me thinking that was how I had to be around boys and men. I live with a man and have two children but I have had relationships with three women. I am very confused about my sexuality. LESLEY-LEIGH

> I am ashamed of my own body. I never liked undressing in front of anyone; at school I would be caned because I refused to change for gym or get a shower. I am unable to relax and enjoy sex with my wife. I have no interest in sex at all. GRAHAM

It is difficult to work on sexual difficulties until you have worked on the problems resulting from the other three processes described below. Sexual difficulties are not specifically covered in this book but are discussed in *Breaking Free*.

Stigmatization

Some children who are sexually abused may believe for a time that what is happening to them is 'normal'. However, at some point most child victims feel the abuse is wrong and shameful even when they don't understand exactly what is happening. Abusers may blame children for the abuse, tell them to keep the abuse secret and frighten them into silence. This secrecy makes children feel that there is something to feel guilty and ashamed about. Other people who are told or find out about the abuse may be shocked and blame the victim or put pressure on him or her to remain silent. This can add to the feeling of shame. Adult Survivors often continue to keep the secret for fear of other people's reactions and because they feel ashamed.

As a result of the process of stigmatization many Survivors blame themselves for the abuse and may also feel responsible and guilty for anything bad that happens to them or to other people they know. Survivors have told us they feel 'dirty' and ashamed because of the things that have been done to them. Survivors often feel bad about themselves and different from other people. They may therefore isolate themselves from other people and avoid making close friendships. The feelings of shame and guilt can lead Survivors to abuse and punish themselves with drugs, alcohol or through self-mutilation and suicide attempts. Some Survivors feel so different that they see themselves as outsiders in society, unable to care about what happens to them or what they do. Survivors who feel like this may start to behave in criminal or anti-social ways and end up in court or prison.

Write down any of your problems which result from stigmatization:

_____

_____

_____

_____

_____

_____

_____

Examples

> I used to get involved in dangerous games like playing with fire, jumping out of windows in high buildings, and hitch-hiking. I'd numbed myself from my abuse, had no sense of danger and didn't care about my safety. My abusers didn't respect or care about me so I didn't believe I was important either. SARAH

> The abuse has made me very critical of myself and I cannot accept myself. I find it difficult to accept a 'pat on the back' and feel people are just being kind, not that I've done something to deserve praise. ANITA B

> I have had drink and drug problems – it's a nice feeling to forget for a while. LESLEY-LEIGH

> I feel ashamed and unclean. I have a problem with cleanliness; I brush my teeth about eight times a day and I never feel satisfied that the house is clean enough. GRAHAM

Chapters 5–7 are designed to help you work on the feelings of guilt and shame resulting from stigmatization.

Betrayal

When children are abused, especially by relatives or someone they know or like, their trust is betrayed. Abusers often build up trusting relationships with children and may make them feel wanted and cared for before abusing them. They manipulate the trust and vulnerability of children and disregard their well-being. Child and adult Survivors may also feel betrayed by non-abusing mothers, family, friends and professionals who do not support and protect them.

Betrayal can be experienced as a feeling of loss – loss of a trusting and loving relationship – and this can lead to feelings of grief and depression, or anger and hostility. Fear of betrayal can also lead to mistrust of others and cause Survivors to withdraw or feel uncomfortable in close relationships. On the other hand, some Survivors become extremely dependent and clingy. Being betrayed by the very people one would expect to be able to trust can result in Survivors having difficulties in trusting other people. They may not be able to trust or they may have difficulties knowing who can be trusted. This in turn makes the Survivors vulnerable to further abuse and exploitation, especially if they are unable to judge trustworthiness or feel compelled to cling on to bad relationships.

Write down any of your problems which result from betrayal:

_____

_____

_____

_____

_____

_____

_____

Examples

I find it hard to have friendships. I find it hard to trust people, I always think they are lying to me. I find it hard to show my children love but you cannot show love if you have never been shown it. I'm learning how to do this. LESLEY-LEIGH

I feel angry towards people and I don't trust many people. I am over-protective towards my children and won't let them stay overnight at a friend's house. PAULA

Chapters 8 and 9 help you begin to work on issues of betrayal by exploring your relationships with your abusers and with your mothers or other non-abusing care-givers.

Powerlessness

Children experience an intense sense of powerlessness during sexual abuse. Children's bodies are touched or invaded and this may happen again and again. Abusers manipulate children and may physically force them into abuse. Children feel powerless to stop the abuse or reveal what is happening. Even when children do tell they may not be believed. Children repeatedly experience fear and an inability to control the situation.

The powerlessness experienced in sexual abuse can lead to long-term feelings of being unable to take action or change situations. Survivors thus feel powerless to prevent further abuse and may end up feeling like victims all their lives. Feeling powerless and out of control can produce panic attacks, anxiety, phobias and nightmares. Survivors may try to escape from their fears and feelings of powerlessness by running away from home or from school, or by withdrawing emotionally. Emotional withdrawal can take the form of depression, blanking out or blacking out, or living in a fantasy world. Survivors may also react to feeling powerless by attempting to take control and by making themselves feel more powerful in some way. Eating disorders often involve a desperate attempt to exert some control, by controlling one's food intake and body weight. Obsessive-compulsive behaviours such as excessive counting, checking or cleaning can also be ways of coping with feeling out of control. Some Survivors try to feel more powerful by aggressive behaviour, by bullying, being abusive or by controlling other people.

Write down any of your problems which result from powerlessness:

_____

_____

_____

_____

_____

_____

_____

Examples

The problems I have which result from feeling powerless are: flashbacks, phobias, anxiety, feeling like a victim, obsessed with cleaning, needing to be in control. PAULA

I feel weak and unimportant and find it difficult to make decisions. I experience flashbacks, hallucinations, bad dreams and panic attacks. GRAHAM

Chapter 7 helps you see that you have more power now than you did when you were a child. Chapter 8 aims to help you feel more empowered in relation to your abuser.

Survivor's comment

I found it hard to keep in control of my feelings when I was doing this exercise. I had flashbacks, my mind wandered off to what happened. I was scared and angry and wanted revenge on my abusers. I calmed myself down by telling

> myself I am in control now. It also helped to have someone in the room with me who understood what I have been through and I went back to Chapter 1 and looked at the ways I could look after myself. PAULA

Childhood abuse is a traumatic event that has many different effects on the lives of Survivors. Some of the effects are a direct result of the abuse, such as feeling guilty, having flashbacks or hallucinations, being confused about your sexual orientation or identity, being over-protective of children, feeling depressed or having problems trusting other people. Other problems arise indirectly as a result of the ways Survivors cope with the abuse. When people feel bad or have bad experiences they have to find some way of coping with them. Survivors often cope with their memories and feelings about the abuse by drinking alcohol, keeping busy, working hard, cutting themselves, eating a lot or pushing their memories away. Nearly all of these coping strategies start off as useful ways of coping with bad experiences but some can develop into problems themselves.

Many Survivors see their current problems as signs that there is something wrong with them or that they are bad people, rather than understanding that the problems may be a result of the abuse or of the creative ways they have used to cope with and survive the abuse. The next exercise asks you to think about your past and current problems and to try to relate them to your past experiences. This is to help you understand that your symptoms were a response to how you were feeling and what was happening to you at different times in your life.

EXERCISE 2.5   HOW THE ABUSE HAS AFFECTED MY LIFE

Aim   To help you look at your past and current problems and to relate them to your abusive experiences.

1 Think about yourself at different ages from childhood to the present. Remember what was happening to you at these times and try to relate your symptoms and problems to your experiences. Remember that some of the problems will have resulted from the way you were treated (e.g. feeling bad about yourself or flashbacks) and others will be ways you tried to survive and cope with your feelings (e.g. self-harm or working too hard).
2 Write an account of the kinds of difficulties you have experienced and how you think they relate to the abuse.

The example that follows may help you. Some of you may prefer to draw a diagram or use one of the other alternatives to writing.

How the abuse has affected my life

Catherine's example

I always felt different to other children but I didn't know why at the time. The abuse had made me feel unworthy which made it hard for me to make friends. I felt aggressive to younger children and any friends I did manage to make. If I hadn't been abused I wouldn't have grown up feeling different to other children and I wouldn't have felt like no one liked me or wanted to be my friend. I had a poor self-image.

Later on, in adolescence, my low self-esteem made me feel ugly and I used to worry that no boy would ever be interested in me. Because of what the abuse taught me I let boys use my body without respect for me. When I was 15 I remember having a bag of broken glass, hidden under my bed, at the ready. I slashed my arms up to get rid of the emotional pain I couldn't understand. I also remember drinking bottles of wine on my own at that age.

Life at university was a nightmare. Being away from the abusive situation was opportunity for my emotions to surface. I was very mixed up and I started with anorexia nervosa then with bulimia nervosa. I was socially inept. I lived on my own in a rented room and I had no friends. It was three years of hell. I buried myself in my work – it was all I knew how to do.

Later on I had relationship problems – lads could do what they liked with me – why ever not? It was what I had learnt from the abuser – I was there for others, not for me. I suffered difficulties in my marriage. I was emotionally demanding, clingy and very dependent. I could not return the physical love my husband offered, I thought this was something he did to me and I was conditioned into blanking out whenever things got intimate. The slashing and other self-injury started again. If I hadn't been abused I wouldn't have suffered the bouts of depression, the feelings of despair and nothingness, time after time. There was some new problem every six months or so. Always something round the corner to halt any growth in my self-esteem and confidence.

Looking to the future

This is how Rebecca described her problems at the beginning of therapy:

The abuse has greatly affected my life. My childhood was lost and I now experience depression, anger, frustration and constant fear. I feel that I am totally worthless, useless and have no right to live. It has destroyed my ability to love and care and left me with a compulsive need to be in control of everything and everyone. I feel afraid I will abuse other people to gain that control. I hate myself, my body and my spirit because I am evil and rotten through and through. I don't think I will ever be able to experience a full relationship with someone and that makes me angry. I want to hurt myself all the time.

Rebecca now writes:

The writing above, was how I felt when I came into therapy. Some of the problems were not due to the sexual abuse but to other experiences in my childhood. It makes me feel very sad to see how I was so obviously very deeply depressed and could not see any hope at all. I now realize just how far I have come. The changes have been subtle and not always easy to see. I don't self-injure anymore. The depression I have lived with all my life has begun to take a back seat. I don't wish I was dead anymore. That has to be good. Today I feel generally well. I am now very close to discontinuing my anti-depressant medication which I have taken for the last five years. My mood swings are less severe and very much less frequent. I have learned to talk about how I am feeling which is the most positive improvement. I have also learned to laugh and cry – emotions I found difficult to express before. I no longer blame myself for the abuse I suffered and I no longer immediately blame myself if things go wrong. It is getting easier to have relationships and I am moving towards those relationships (sexual) that for me are most fraught with difficulty. My friendships are more equal and productive. I generally feel good about myself and my body. This is not true every day, but who feels good all the time? My life is very different now, I can hold down a job (a good professional position) and I am able to make plans for my future career. I am even planning to commence a degree course in the next year. Today the world looks very different. I am more optimistic about my future and I have achieved what I set out to do – to feel content and satisfied with who I am.

You have looked back at what has happened to you in the past and seen the range of problems resulting from your experiences. It may be that some of your problems are related to experiences in your life other than the sexual abuse. It is hard to known which problems are caused by the abuse and impossible to know what you would be like now if you hadn't been abused. What is possible, though, is to work on your current problems and to take some control of the way your life goes from now on. You are already moving towards this by working through this book.

Becoming aware of the extent of your problems can be very distressing. The problems you have may be a result of the abuse or how you learnt to cope with your painful experiences. Remind yourself that it is normal to have problems when you have experienced abuse or trauma and, like Rebecca, you can begin to overcome them. The next chapter helps you to understand more about the coping strategies you use and also helps you to begin replacing harmful coping strategies with less harmful ones.

Before you move on notice how you are feeling now and take care of yourself.

3
Coping Strategies

Everybody has to find ways to cope when they are faced by problems, bad experiences, and painful feelings. If we are able to, we might confide in someone else, try to solve the problem, seek help and advice, or comfort and look after ourselves. When children are sexually abused, however, they usually cannot speak out or stop what is happening and there may be nowhere to go for comfort and support. They have to find *some* way to cope and to survive and so they often try to block out thoughts and feelings about the abuse as a way of trying to control the emotional pain they are in. Blocking can be a very necessary survival strategy in situations where there is no escape. However, for many Survivors blocking becomes a habit that is carried into adult life and can create problems in the long term.

This chapter helps you to understand more about the coping strategies that, consciously or unconsciously, you currently use to deal with painful memories and feelings about being sexually abused. Some of your strategies may be causing you harm and we encourage you to begin to find less harmful ways of coping and to use your strategies with more awareness. We start by looking at blocking strategies that are commonly used by Survivors and then at expressing and processing strategies that are more helpful in the long term. The exercises in this chapter and the rest of the book help you move towards expressing and processing your thoughts and feelings rather than blocking them off.

Types of coping strategies

Blocking strategies

There are many different strategies that can be used to block out memories and feelings or to distract one's focus of attention from them. Alcohol, drugs and food are often used as ways of trying to forget problems and to alter how you feel. Unfortunately, if they are used in excess they can be harmful and leave you with a further problem. Keeping busy, going out all the time, cleaning, checking, compulsively caring for others, sleeping or self-harming until the physical pain becomes greater than the emotional pain can also serve the same purpose. These ways of coping often become automatic responses to distressing feelings and problems. Survivors may not consciously understand why they are doing these things and sometimes start to believe that they must be 'mad' or 'bad'. Coping strategies that block memories and feelings are problematic in that they never resolve the underlying difficulty and they may go on to become problems in their own right, such as an addiction or obsession. However, some of these strategies can be useful if used in moderation and as a short-term measure, for example, to take a break from difficulties or to allow you to complete certain tasks such as going to work.

Dissociation

Dissociation is a strategy that many Survivors use as children and as adults to escape from their painful thoughts and feelings. They separate part of themselves off from what is happening and from their distress and pain. Some children describe stepping outside their bodies and watching themselves being abused without experiencing any of the physical and emotional pain. Others invent a fantasy world into which they can retreat every time they are being abused. Some Survivors create different parts of themselves to hold different memories and feelings and to cope with different situations.

> The hurt started when I was about three years old when my dad started to come into the bathroom to wash my hair. His excuse was that he had to check that I had washed myself down there. I told my mum he was hurting me but I did not tell her how he was hurting me. She insisted that he kept washing my hair. I had to forget the hurt so I used to switch off and talk to a friend inside myself that I had created. Her name was 'Baby' and she took most of the hurt. JEAN

Dissociation is a way in which children cope with continuing to be abused and in which adult Survivors cut off from the painful thoughts and memories about the abuse. Many Survivors who dissociate are not aware of how much they are doing this.

Expressing and processing strategies

The exercises in this book ask you to take a different approach to dealing with your pain. They ask you to write, to talk, to paint or to use other non-verbal ways of expressing yourself. Instead of blocking or distracting from your feelings and memories they help you to experience and express them and to learn to think and feel in a new way about your past.

> The exercises helped me to get in touch with my feelings and break through

my denial and minimization. They also helped me release pent-up emotions in appropriate ways. SARAH

As a child you were probably unable to express your thoughts and feelings about the abuse directly because you had to keep it secret. This was not right and as an adult you can choose to do something different. Writing, talking, and painting are non-harmful coping strategies that you can learn to use in your everyday life not just when you are doing these exercises. Some people find it helps to keep a journal to note down their feelings day by day. Survivors have also recommended dancing, singing, sculpting and listening to music as ways of getting in touch with and releasing their feelings.

Self-care and support strategies

We also want to encourage you to understand more about what you want and need and to seek comfort and support from others and to learn to look after yourself. Some strategies such as walking in the countryside or having a massage are ways of looking after yourself, strengthening yourself physically and emotionally, and balancing painful and difficult work with reminding yourself of the positive things in life. When you were sexually abused your physical and emotional needs were ignored. You may have also learned ways to block off from your feelings and to numb the physical pain you were in. All these things can set off a pattern of not caring for yourself and not attending to your own needs.

Coping strategies often become automatic reactions to feelings and difficulties. You may not always be aware of what is happening or why you feel compelled to act in a certain way. Behaviours can have many different functions and cannot always be put into one category – blocking or expressing and processing or self-care and support. Sleeping, for example, can be a way of blocking off and also a way of looking after yourself.

The series of exercises below are designed to help you become aware of what strategies you are currently using and why, and to strengthen your use of expressing and self-care strategies.

EXERCISE 3.1   IDENTIFYING YOUR COPING STRATEGIES

Aim   To look at the different ways you deal with feelings, memories and problems.

Below is a list of different ways that people cope with feelings, memories and problems. Look at the list and for each strategy rate how frequently you use it by putting a tick under one of the columns. Add to the list any other ways you cope with difficulties and rate how often you use these strategies. Some of these strategies (e.g. self-harm) could be problems in themselves but for the moment record all the strategies you use whether or not they are problematic.

	Often	Sometimes	Hardly ever	Never	Used to but don't now
Cleaning (house or self)					
Sleeping					
Keeping busy					
Going out a lot					
Staying in a lot					
Blanking off feelings					
Fantasizing/ daydreaming					
Dissociating/cutting off					
Passing out					
Taking medication					
Drinking alcohol					
Taking non-prescribed drugs					
Smoking					
Self-harming					
Withdrawing from other people					
Over-eating/binge-eating					
Under-eating/starving					
Working on computer					
Working					
Suicide attempts					
Becoming aggressive					
Having a bath					
Resting					
Painting how I feel					
Writing					
Phoning someone					
Talking to someone					
Walking					
Having a massage					
Exercising					
Dancing					
Listening to music					
Reading					

	Often	Sometimes	Hardly ever	Never	Used to but don't now

Survivors' comments

I realized how much I do when I am trying to cope with things. LESLEY-LEIGH

It enabled me to look seriously at all the coping strategies I either engage in or had engaged in previously. I was quite shocked to see how many I used. It is important to see things as they really are in order to get better. REBECCA

Benefits and problems of coping strategies

As we have seen there are many different strategies that can be used to deal with feelings and difficulties. Some strategies, for example writing a journal, may be entirely helpful and cause you no additional problems. Other strategies although helpful can also have their problems or downsides or may be helpful if used in moderation but cause further problems if used in excess.

I started to drink alcohol to block out my feelings about the abuse. I thought it would be an escape for me; however, it never was – it only made me worse. It resulted in me getting into trouble with the authorities, i.e. police, courts, the justice system etc. My behaviour led me to receiving probation orders and also curfews and being barred from all public houses and off-licences. These restrictions only aggravated the way I was feeling, leading me to abuse alcohol even more, i.e. drinking at home and finding other areas where I could drink like Leeds where I was unknown to the police. I have also ended up in mental institutions over the years and been admitted to detox for six weeks which helped a little but did not stop me from drinking because I still had deep feelings about the abuse. ANTHONY

Anthony started to drink alcohol when he was 15. Initially he had found drinking a moderate amount of alcohol a useful coping strategy as it helped him block out his memories and feelings about being abused. Over time, however, Anthony developed a problem with alcohol itself – he became physically and psychologically dependent on it and got into trouble when he was drunk. Eventually Anthony had a number of other problems to cope with in addition to the abuse and he began to see the downside of alcohol as a coping strategy.

Anthony joined a Survivors' group and began to understand more about his feelings and experiences and to develop less harmful ways of coping.

> I have not been in any real trouble since starting therapy. I no longer blame myself for being abused and I do not bottle things up or keep things to myself any more. I have more control over myself and my life now in general is much better. ANTHONY

Sarah, Paula and Lesley-Leigh have also learnt more about their ways of coping and can see how their strategies help but can also cause problems.

> I cope by blanking off my feelings. It helps me at the time but then my feelings catch up with me and I over-react. It also makes it hard to do anything about a situation when the impact doesn't hit you until later. SARAH

> Eating chocolate calms my nerves but in the long run I just want more chocolate to forget other things. PAULA

> Although keeping busy takes my mind off my feelings I sometimes don't have time for my family. LESLEY-LEIGH

EXERCISE 3.2   BENEFITS AND PROBLEMS OF YOUR COPING STRATEGIES

Aim   To understand how your coping strategies help you and how they might also cause problems.

Write down the coping strategies you use under the first column. Think about how each coping strategy helps and write this down under the second column. Now think about what problems (if any) might result from this strategy and record this under column three. It might help you to look at Rebecca's example at the end of the exercise.

Coping strategy	How it helps	Downside/problems
Examples		
Drinking alcohol	Helps me forget the abuse. Makes me feel more confident	Doesn't solve the problem. Addiction. More problems when I'm drunk
Cutting self	Relieves tension. Changes emotional pain to physical pain	Scars I can't get rid of. Embarrassed when people see them

Rebecca's example

Rebecca's example is recorded in full so you can see the range of coping strategies one person might have and follow her example through to Exercise 3.3.

Coping strategy	How it helps	Downside/problems
Bathing	Relieves tension. Gives space to think	None
Resting	Gives space to think	Can be just a way of escaping
Cleaning	Physical release of tension. Sense of achievement	Can become an obsession if taken too far. OK in moderation

Coping strategy	How it helps	Downside/problems
Painting	Release of emotional pain and expression of feeling	None
Writing	Can make order out of confusion. Naming of feelings. Gives some focus for solution	None
Sleeping	Escape from emotional pain	Pain still has to be faced on waking
Keeping busy	No time to dwell on problem	OK in moderation. Can become a way to avoid the problem or feelings
Staying in	Avoids other problems and people	Leads to further depression, bad feelings and difficulty in communicating
Medication	Reduces physical and emotional pain	None in moderation. Can lead to psychological and physical dependency
Distracting	Takes mind off difficulty	None as long as difficulty is not ignored
Drinking alcohol	Reduces anxiety, dulls feelings	In excess leads to dependency, and physical problems
Becoming aggressive	Reduces tension	Depression. Damage to others and to property
Withdrawing from others	Gives physical space to think	Cuts down possibility of looking at difficulty objectively and isolates
Over-eating/ bingeing	Quick way of suppressing anxiety and bad feeling	Health and weight difficulties. Makes me feel unattractive. Low self-esteem
Under-eating/starving	Greater feeling of self-control	Illness. False sense of control

Coping strategy	How it helps	Downside/problems
Phone/talk to someone	Sharing difficulty. Gain support. Relieve feelings of anxiety	None unless you expect others to solve the problem
Exercise	Relieves tension. Feeling of achievement	None in moderation
Working on computer	Relieves tension. Moves focus from feeling or problem	None as long as it's not used as a long-term escape
Sculpture	Achievement. Relieves anxiety. Focuses attention on expression of feelings	None

Survivors' comments

> It took time to think about each strategy and how they made me feel. I don't think I have ever spent time on this level of analysis. It helped me to see strategies that were helpful and unhelpful and how. I felt that I still use a lot of negative/unhelpful ways of coping. I was sad that this was the case but I accepted them. I was also able to identify a few of the good strategies that I had developed. REBECCA

> By doing this exercise I realized that the things I do have some reason. LESLEY-LEIGH

It is important for all of us to have coping strategies to use at difficult times. Some coping strategies are harmless, some are harmless if used in moderation, and some coping strategies can be harmful and go on to become problems in their own right. It is obviously better to try to use coping strategies which will not cause you further harm. In the short term, however, you may have difficulty in not using harmful coping strategies. Don't worry about this; at the moment you are only trying to become more aware of how your coping strategies help and how they cause problems.

EXERCISE 3.3   WHICH OF YOUR COPING STRATEGIES ARE HARMFUL?

Aim   To sort out which strategies are non-harmful and which strategies are generally harmful, or harmful if used in excess.

Refer back to how you described each of your coping strategies in exercise 3.2 and now sort them into the three categories below. Use your own judgement about whether the strategies are harmful or not. Different people will judge their own strategies in different ways.

Non-harmful

_____

_____

_____

_____

_____

Harmless in moderation but harmful in excess

_____

_____

_____

_____

Generally harmful or problematic

_____

_____

_____

_____

Examples

Rebecca

Non-harmful

Bathing	Phone someone
Painting	Talk to someone
Writing	Working on computer
Sculpture	

Harmless in moderation but harmful in excess

Exercising	Keeping busy
Distracting	Medication
Resting	Cleaning
Sleeping	

Generally harmful or problematic

Staying in	Over-eating/bingeing
Drinking alcohol	Under-eating/starving
Becoming aggressive	Withdrawal from others

Wakefield Survivors' Moving On Group

Non-harmful

Bathing	Dancing
Resting	Listening to music
Writing	Phoning someone
Drawing	Talking to someone

Harmless in moderation but harmful in excess

Sleeping	Distracting
Taking medication	Withdrawing from other people
Exercising	Working hard
Keeping busy	Playing the joker
Blanking off feelings	Listening to other people's problems

Generally harmful or problematic

Self-harming	Lashing out at others
Smoking	Pretending the abuse didn't happen

Survivors' comments

I found the exercise very helpful. It enabled me to categorize these coping strategies and see where I was. It was difficult to decide which fitted into which category but I assessed where they should go for me personally. I completed the exercise at a time when I was having to rely on these strategies to survive. I became quite concerned when I realized that some of the things that I felt were helping at that moment were not, and that it was difficult to access the strategies that were non-harmful. REBECCA

I know some things are harmful like smoking or not eating or taking too many tablets – harmful for the body. But some things, like crying and talking, I feel are bad because I have been told not to do them. BRONWYN

It made me realize how many positive ways there are to cope instead of using negative ones. Be as honest as you can about how you cope and whether it is negative or positive, e.g. starving is a negative way of coping although sometimes if I am losing weight it seems positive and a good idea at the time. CORAL

I admitted to myself that I do some things that are harmful. LESLEY-LEIGH

EXERCISE 3.4   MY LIST OF NON-HARMFUL COPING STRATEGIES
Aim   To have a ready-made list of non-harmful coping strategies to refer to in times of difficulty.

List below all the helpful and non-harmful coping strategies you can think of, including those in exercise 3.3. You do not have to be currently using these strategies to list them here. Ask other people what they do to cope with feeling bad and list the strategies here if you think they are useful and non-harmful.

Non-harmful coping strategies

_____

_____

_____

_____

_____

_____

_____

_____

Example
Wakefield Survivors' Group positive/non-harmful coping strategies

Taking things one step at a time	Seeing it as it was
Writing a letter	Meditation
Taking some time out	Laughing
Looking after yourself	Playing
Talking/sharing your feelings	Healing tears
Ripping up an old phone book	Dancing
Massage/body work	Singing
Respecting and loving myself	Walking

Hitting/thumping/throwing objects without hurting yourself

Pausing/delaying – finding out what you are feeling and who you are feeling it about

Going to the doctor and getting further help and advice

Survivor's comment

> It was easy to complete from my list in Exercise 3.3 but I found it difficult to
> ask others how they coped. I found people I trusted and respected to add
> things to my list. REBECCA

Strengthening your use of non-harmful coping strategies

During the next week try to use the non-harmful coping strategies on your list. To begin using non-harmful coping strategies and to maintain their use you need to become aware of what difficulties you are having day by day and what coping strategies you are using. It can be very tempting to return to old familiar ways of coping. Notice when you are doing this and if possible substitute a non-harmful coping strategy at least once during the week. Gradually begin to try to use ways of expressing and processing your feelings rather than blocking or distracting yourself. Sometimes, however, you may need to block or distract to stop yourself feeling overwhelmed and give yourself some time out from this work. Try to use the least harmful strategy to do this. Don't worry if you use old harmful coping strategies – this does not mean you have failed. At this stage you're trying to become aware of what you are doing and why you are doing it. Changing old habits takes longer. Coping strategies which have become problems in their own right such as alcohol or drug use, eating disorders and self-harm may require you to seek professional help. But it is never too soon to try to make some changes, however small.

EXERCISE 3.5   MONITORING COPING STRATEGIES
Aim   To help you focus on the kinds of coping strategies you are using day by day as a first step to increasing the use of helpful and non-harmful strategies.

During the next week fill in the table below. Each day record any difficult feelings or problems you experience in column 1 and then in column 2 record what coping strategies you used to try to deal with each of these difficulties. Record all your attempts to deal with your difficulties irrespective of how harmful or harmless they are. Try to fill this in as near as possible to the time you experienced the difficulty. You might want to make your own copies of the table so that you can repeat this exercise from time to time whilst you are working through this book.

	Difficulty	Coping strategies
Examples	Had a row Felt angry and upset	Binged on chocolate Phoned a friend
Monday		
Tuesday		
Wednesday		
Thursday		
Friday		
Saturday		
Sunday		

Rebecca's example

	Difficulty	Coping strategies
Monday	Great difficulty at work. Felt afraid and vulnerable	Withdrew. Took extra medication. Inadequate eating. Went for a massage
Tuesday	Continuation of yesterday's difficulties. Felt afraid and vulnerable, also angry and responsible	Talked it through with my therapist. Put difficulty into perspective. Cuddled my purple cushion (my safety object)

	Difficulty	Coping strategies
Wednesday	Feeling frightened and stressed	Talked to colleagues and boss about the situation and gained their support. Tried to shut off how I had handled the situation. Came close to 'shut down' (non-functioning) but knew this wasn't the answer. It would only have made the problem worse
Thursday	Anxious because work not done for tomorrow. Angry that other things had led to distraction and now I had to do it on my day off	Writing down how I felt. Planned out action I needed to take. Got on with it and sacrificed day off to reduce anxiety
Friday	Felt inadequate as a professional and a person	Made a list of feelings about my job and put them into fact and fiction columns – I was therefore able to see exactly what was true and what was imagined. Then distracted myself
Saturday	No real difficulty	
Sunday	Felt battered and tired	Finished this exercise. Returned to earlier affirmation writings and realized just how much better things were

Survivor's comment

It helped me look logically at a problem instead of catastrophizing. It also helped me identify individual feelings whereas I often just have a blanket depressed feeling. As the week moved on I felt more enlightened and slowed down. I kept on completing the exercise and it helped me see reality. I think it will help me to focus on using positive coping mechanisms when difficulties arise. REBECCA

Giving yourself positive experiences

When we are feeling very depressed, fearful or confused it can become difficult to remember the things we usually do that make us happy or at least help to maintain us on an even keel. We need to make sure that every day we do some of the things that will help maintain our well-being.

EXERCISE 3.6   GIVING YOURSELF POSITIVE EXPERIENCES

Aim   To make sure you give yourself positive experiences and start the day in a positive frame of mind by reminding yourself that there are things that give you pleasure.

1   Each morning when you wake up, before you have opened your eyes, think of three things that you are going to do today that you will like. They don't have to be big things. They can be small, everyday things e.g. drinking a cup of coffee, having a bath or watching your favourite TV programme.
2   When you are in a good mood write a list below of ten things that give you pleasure. Try to do one of these things each day.

Ten things I enjoy

-
-

-
-

-
-

-
-

-
-

Example
Annabelle's way of giving herself pleasurable experiences

Pick some flowers	Paint my toenails
Have a day out on the train	Do a crossword
Read a book	Go to bed early
Tune into a different radio channel	Plant some bulbs
Go for a walk/swim	Hire a video
Enrol in a night class	Buy a plant
Go to the cinema	Make a picnic and go out for the day

In this chapter we have tried to help you learn more about the strategies you use to cope with the effects of being abused. You may be using blocking strategies which are harmful or have become problems themselves. We hope you can now try to use more of the non-harmful coping strategies to understand, express and process your experiences. Looking after yourself, and thinking about and doing things you enjoy are also positive ways to help you cope. At times you may feel that you still need to use old harmful coping strategies. This does not mean you have failed or 'gone back to square one'. It takes time to change long-term habits, especially if they feel familiar and safe. In the next chapter we continue to help you cope with your difficulties by looking at how memories and feelings are triggered and what you can do about this.

4
Dealing with Emotions, Flashbacks and Hallucinations

Sexual abuse is a traumatic experience and often recurs time and time again. Children can find this experience so overwhelming that they are unable to process and come to terms with their thoughts and feelings about what is happening. As adults, Survivors can continue to be troubled by unprocessed memories and feelings. They may feel continually flooded and overwhelmed or they may try to cope by blocking off. In the last chapter we looked at the many different coping strategies that can be used to block off thoughts and feelings, some of which can go on to become problems in their own right. Pushing away memories and feelings can be a very useful and necessary thing to do at times. However, one of the difficulties with this strategy is that there are many things which might remind you of your abuse and you may not always be able to avoid them. Survivors who try to push away their memories and feelings are vulnerable to being suddenly reminded of the abuse. This can result in extreme emotional states, flashbacks and hallucinations.

This chapter helps you to understand more about what triggers emotional states, flashbacks and hallucinations and to find ways of beginning to get some control over these experiences. To overcome these symptoms you will need to continue to work on the underlying trauma – the sexual abuse – but for now you may be able to get a little more control over what can be very frightening and confusing experiences.

Extreme emotional states, flashbacks and hallucinations

Extreme emotional states
Extreme emotional states can result from the triggering of past experiences. Painful feelings can come flooding back. Panic attacks, bouts of depression, fits of rage or floods of tears for no apparent reason are frequently described by Survivors. You may be taken by surprise by your feelings and be unable to

45

understand where they are coming from and what they are about. You may not feel much about your own abuse but find yourself weeping profusely at a film or book, or being mad with rage at an injustice that has been done to another person. You may find yourself being angry at people for what appears on the surface to be trivial reasons.

Flashbacks

Flashbacks are vivid memories in which a person feels they are re-experiencing past events. During a flashback the Survivor feels as if he or she is a child again and is reliving the abuse. Flashbacks are one of the ways in which blocked off feelings and memories can surface. They can happen at any time or anywhere but are usually triggered off by reminders of the abuse.

> While having sex with my husband he suddenly became the abuser. I pushed him off and jumped out of bed in fear. This was the first time my husband experienced me having a flashback. JEAN

Hallucinations

Many Survivors we have worked with have told us about experiencing the presence of their abuser when they cannot possibly be there. They see their abusers, hear them (often making threats), smell them, sense their presence or feel themselves being abused again.

> I would see my abuser walking towards me with that look in his eyes that told me what he was going to do. I would want to hide in a corner to get away from him. Sometimes I could not see him but I could smell him – the smell on him of the mill where he worked. JEAN

Survivors who have these kind of hallucinations have often been strongly threatened about the consequences of disclosing the abuse.

> My abuser died in 1979 but he had always told me he could come back. After his death I saw him lots of times and I was convinced he had kept his word because he wanted me to keep quiet about the abuse. JEAN

When Survivors experience hallucinations they believe their abuser is really with them in the present and continues to have power and control over them. This is obviously a very frightening experience. It can also be very frightening to see, hear or feel your abuser when you know he or she cannot possibly be there. Survivors sometimes also hallucinate other things.

> The first hallucination happened when I was washing myself and when I looked in the mirror I began to see worm like things crawling under my skin. At the time I was horrified and the fear inside me was overwhelming. It came to the

stage where I would never look at myself in a mirror and my wife had to remove all the mirrors in the house. I believed that my deceased abuser was doing this to make me go insane as a punishment for revealing details of my past. I also sometimes hear my name being called. GRAHAM

Many Survivors think they are going mad and are too frightened to tell anyone about their experiences. Having these kind of experiences is not unusual for Survivors. People who have experienced other traumas such as a bereavement also sometimes experience hallucinations.

Extreme emotional states, flashbacks and hallucinations can be very frightening and undermine your ability to cope. It is therefore important to find ways to understand and control these experiences. The first step towards this is to understand more about what triggers these experiences. The next exercise helps you to do this.

Identifying triggers

A trigger is anything that reminds you of your abuse or brings up feelings associated with the abuse. Triggers often operate out of our awareness or on the edge of our awareness. Triggers can come through any of our senses:

- **Hearing** – e.g. words, accents, music.
- **Vision** – e.g. people, places, clothes, objects.
- **Smell** – e.g. cigarette smoke, aftershave.
- **Touch** – e.g. materials, physical contact.
- **Taste** – e.g. alcohol.

EXERCISE 4.1   IDENTIFYING TRIGGERS
Aim   To identify what triggers emotional states, flashbacks and hallucinations for you.

1   Below is a list of common triggers to emotional states, flashbacks and hallucinations. If you feel able, take a quick look through this list. Some of the words may disturb you and you may find that reading the list acts as a trigger to memories and feelings. If you begin to experience problems or feel you cannot cope, move on to part 2 of the exercise.

Common triggers

Words	Phrases
Parts of the body	I love you
e.g. breast, cock, cunt, bottom	I'm not going to hurt you

Relationship of the abuser to you

e.g. father, mother granddad,
brother, aunty

Sexual words

e.g. sex, suck, fuck

Daddy's little girl

You like this don't you?

Good boy

Smells

Tobacco

Alcohol

Aftershave

Engine oil

Grass

Sweat

Places

Bathroom

Bedroom

Allotment

Garden shed

The house/place where you were
abused

The town where you were abused

Sexual behaviours

Oral sex

Masturbation

Certain sexual positions
e.g. someone on top of you

Anal intercourse

Types of touch, e.g. stroking

Kissing

Being looked at

People

Your abuser

Children

Someone who looks like your abuser

Someone who has the same job/role
as your abuser e.g. vicar, doctor,
caretaker

Someone who acts or talks in the
same way as your abuser

Clothes

Jeans

Shorts

Bathrobe

Pyjamas

Underwear

Uniforms

Clothes made of certain material
e.g. crimplene, nylon, silk,
cotton

Situations

Arguments

Feeling trapped

Feeling rejected

Feeling powerless

Feeling betrayed

Feeling ignored/unheard

Other

Glazed eyes	Tickling
False teeth	Sitting next to someone
Nakedness	A certain time of day, e.g. evening
Pubic hair	A certain day of the week
Certain types of music	A certain time of the year,
Alcohol	e.g. Christmas
Drugs	Photographs
Chocolate	Weather, e.g. wind, rain, sun
Media reports of abuse	Lack of sleep
	Certain tastes

2 Under each heading below write down anything which you *know* is a trigger for you, or which you think *might be* a trigger for you. Use the above list to help you. You will also probably be able to think of many other triggers that aren't included here. Write them down if you are able to but don't worry if this is too difficult at the moment. Keep the list and as you become aware of other triggers write those down too.

Words   **Phrases**

Smells   **Places**

Sexual behaviour   **People**

Clothes   Situations

Others

Jean's example

Words

Abuse

Rape

Dad

Secret

Sex

Bathroom

Phrases

I love you

Do you love me?

Favourite little girl

Can you keep a secret?

Do you like it?

Smells

Cigarettes

Mill-work smell

Sweat

Beer

Places

Bathroom

Bedroom

Toilet

Sexual behaviour

Touching (breast, vagina)

Being stared at

Sometimes just touching (cuddle, putting arms around shoulder)

People

Sisters

Brothers

Someone who looks like my abuser or mother

Clothes

Short skirts

Low-cut tops

Swimwear

Situations

Being trapped in a confined space
with men

Parents kissing daughters

Going to the ladies toilets when the
men's is next door and a man goes
in

Others

Drunks

Photos of when I was little

Hearing about abuse on TV/radio

Watching love scenes on TV

Friends talking about their childhood

Getting dressed/undressed in front of
my husband

Strangers (men) sitting next to me

Survivors' comments

I had not realized the amount of things that got thoughts going in my mind and caused a lot of fears about my abuse. JEAN

This exercise made me think and I felt my mind was more organized when I re-read it. Stick at it. It does work. Try it and see. MAYA

It was good to recognize what I think triggers me off. I still couldn't write down some of the triggers as they reminded me of the abuse. I made a decision not to write down the really difficult stuff. I made a mental note of them so I could deal with them later. Only do what feels comfortable. Pin the list up somewhere private and add to it over several weeks. REBECCA

I didn't realize until now how having my feelings ignored in the present makes me extremely angry. CATHERINE

I started to remember things I had blocked out. You need to be prepared for this. LESLEY-LEIGH

Do not rush the exercise. Think about it carefully. Keep returning to the exercise as more things become apparent. CORAL

For years my husband did the ironing because if I did it I'd feel miserable and anxious and become absorbed in the unhappy relationship I have with my father. Then I had a flashback in which my father had come into my bedroom with his shirt over his head and sleeves flapping pretending to be a ghost. In another flashback I was raped whilst putting freshly laundered sheets and shirts away in the airing cupboard and wardrobe. This made me realize where the anxiety was coming from. I was trying to protect myself from being abused like that again but I no longer need to be on full alert. So now I've no excuse for avoiding doing the ironing! ANNABELLE

Monitoring triggers

It can sometimes be difficult to identify triggers to emotional states, flashbacks and hallucinations. The triggers might be things you have reacted to so often, or so suddenly that you have lost awareness of what they are. The exercises in this chapter aim to bring the triggers back into your awareness.

Persevere with trying to identify the triggers. Try to think back to the point just before you had a flashback or hallucination or started to feel bad. Recall what happened next:

- Where were you?
- What could you see, hear, smell, feel and taste?
- What people were around?
- What was said and done?
- What were you thinking about?

If you were watching the TV or listening to the radio, recall what was happening in the programme you were listening to or watching.

Thoughts that act as triggers can be very difficult to identify because we are constantly thinking and running a commentary on whatever we are doing. Certain trains of thought may have happened so frequently that they become automatic, that is, you are thinking things without really being aware of what you are thinking. These automatic thoughts are important because they can have a profound effect on how you feel. However, when you are not aware of your automatic thoughts it may seem as if your feelings have come 'out of the blue'.

You may experience a panic attack or sense of dread. You might feel weak and start trembling. This is happening for a reason – train yourself to identify the trigger. You might have seen someone who looks like your abuser and it hasn't registered. You might have seen a little girl crying and you start to tremble and want to cry and run away. You might have seen a particular chocolate bar in a shop and you feel sick or sexy. Make yourself stop, concentrate and go back to look carefully for the trigger. Next time you may not be affected or the trigger will be much less potent. ANNABELLE

EXERCISE 4.2 MONITORING TRIGGERS
Aim To focus on a daily basis on what is triggering your emotional states, flashbacks and hallucinations as a first step towards controlling these experiences.

During the next week fill in the table below. Each day record any bad feelings, flashbacks or hallucinations you experience in column 1 and then in column 2 record what you think triggered these experiences. Try to fill this in as near as possible to the time you experienced the problem. Before you start you might want to make copies of these pages so that you can repeat this exercise from time to time whilst you are working through this book.

	Bad feeling, flashbacks, hallucinations	Trigger
Examples	Flashback to being abused aged 7 Felt anxious	Having sex with my partner on top Friends talking about their childhoods
Monday		
Tuesday		
Wednesday		

	Bad feeling, flashbacks, hallucinations	Trigger
Thursday		
Friday		
Saturday		
Sunday		

Maya's example

	Bad feeling, flashbacks, hallucinations	Trigger
Monday	Felt hurt, rejected, a failure as a mother	Not being invited to my daughter's leaving party

	Bad feeling, flashbacks, hallucinations	Trigger
Tuesday	Felt left out, snubbed, upset	Saw a friend with someone else and she ignored me
Wednesday	Felt anxious, insecure	Argued with my husband about children
Thursday	Fear, worry. Flashback to abuse at a young age	A little girl who was playing out alone. She chatted to me and told me her mother was at work
Friday	Fear, dread, guilt, anger. Flashback to finding out my children had been abused whilst I was having a barbecue and enjoying myself	My husband was using the barbecue
Saturday	Envy. Flashback of ill-treatment by my own mother. Upset and confused	Visited a friend and her mother who have a good relationship. Good atmosphere, light-hearted conversation
Sunday	Sad, tearful. Regressed to a young age. Felt sorry for myself. It's not fair	Lying in bed thinking, 'Sundays are family time'

Survivors' comments

I didn't want to spend a week focusing on bad feelings and flashbacks but I knew if I wrote it down I could feel better. It helped me see what was happening and I found it therapeutic. I did pleasurable things during the week as well. MAYA

I suddenly started feeling sad today and I sat and thought about why that was. I was walking my dog and I saw a couple with five children playing games with them. This set me off thinking about my childhood. I can't remember going out with my parents and my sisters and brother, playing football or any other games in the fields as a family. The hurt and pain is all I can remember as a child growing up. I remembered the exercises and about the triggers that can cause you to have flashbacks etc. If I think about it, so many things in life hold memories of some sort like the family in the field – cutting up a cabbage, hearing certain songs, making a mistake when I am driving in my car. JEAN

Dealing with triggers

Identifying your triggers may, in itself, lessen the effect they have on you.

> Sometimes I'd be filled with dread. Then I'd look for the trigger which I had subconsciously registered. Once I had identified it – a little girl in the street, a man smoking a pipe, a graveyard – I seemed to become immune and it wouldn't bother me again. At one time I reached a point where it was almost impossible to go to work because I had become so nervous driving and shook with dread and anxiety along a particular route. Then I looked at a map of the route and there it was! Every morning I had to stop at a zebra crossing and adjacent to it was a street with the same name as the one I'd lived in as a child. Once I realized that, the panic stopped. ANNABELLE

Working on your past abuse by using this book can help you understand and process your experiences and feelings and you will therefore be less likely to suffer sudden emotional states, flashbacks and hallucinations. In the meantime, however, you may also need to find other ways of dealing with the triggers themselves. Below we discuss two ways of doing this – by avoiding them and by using coping strategies.

Avoidance

Some triggers can easily be avoided without interfering with your life too much.

- **Long-term avoidance.** If, for example, you are getting flashbacks during sex and you are able to identify that the triggers are certain positions, acts, types of touch or words that your partner is saying, you could ask your partner not to do or say these things. Think of different things you can do and say to each other that don't remind you of the abuse.
- **Short-term avoidance.** There may be triggers that you would not want to avoid in the long term but could be avoided in the short term as a means of stabilizing your feelings and experiences and gaining a sense of control. Jean found that she often became upset and tearful when trying to relax in the evening and watch TV. She realized that there were often story-lines about children being abused in films and dramas she was watching and that this was triggering her bad feelings. She decided to avoid watching anything about child abuse by turning the TV off or going into another room. Jean hopes this will only need to be a short-term strategy until she feels confident that she can watch these programmes without being badly affected.

EXERCISE 4.3   AVOIDING TRIGGERS
Aim   To help you identify ways in which you could avoid some of your triggers to extreme emotional states, flashbacks and hallucinations.

Under the left-hand column below list any triggers that you think you could avoid without it interfering with your life too much. In the right hand column write a plan of how you are going to avoid the trigger.

Triggers that could be avoided	How to avoid
Jean's example	
Story-lines about child abuse in TV programmes	Turn the TV off or leave the room

_____   _____

_____   _____

_____   _____

_____   _____

_____   _____

_____   _____

_____   _____

_____   _____

Examples

Triggers that could be avoided	How to avoid
Maya	
Staying in bed and feeling depressed. Feeling panicky because I haven't enough time to get things done. Feeling a failure	Make a list of things to do, e.g. get up at 9 a.m. Plan a morning timetable to get work done. Do something enjoyable in the afternoon as a reward
Lesley-Leigh	
Having sex with my partner on top	Find a position that I feel safe in
Seeing my brother	Not going past his house
Certain foods	Do not buy them
Wedding dresses	Do not look at wedding dresses. I won't get married in one

Coral

Certain types of music	Change radio channels to one that is unlikely to play this type of music
Smoky rooms	Open the window
Having photo taken	Don't go places where I am likely to have my photo taken. Tell people I don't want to have my photo taken

Survivor's comment

It made me think about getting out or away from the trigger. Normally I would stay in the situation – I saw this as my punishment. It is going to be hard to put this coping strategy into action but I will try. JEAN

Using coping strategies

Avoiding the things that trigger difficult feelings and experiences is one way of coping. However, you probably cannot avoid all your triggers without severely restricting your life. Once you become aware of what your triggers are, you can start to find other ways of coping. Look back at the non-harmful coping strategies you identified in Exercise 3.4 and think of using one of these coping strategies after a trigger has occurred. Relaxing, challenging your thoughts that something dreadful is going to happen, or using one of your non-harmful coping strategies after you have become aware of a trigger, can stop you going into extreme emotional states or having flashbacks and hallucinations. After the exercise below we suggest some strategies particularly designed to deal with flashbacks and hallucinations.

EXERCISE 4.4   USING COPING STRATEGIES TO DEAL WITH TRIGGERS

Aim   To help you identify coping strategies to deal with your triggers.

List below five triggers that you frequently encounter. For each trigger identify the type of coping strategies you could use in response. Your coping strategies may be different depending on where the trigger occurred, e.g. at home or in a public place.

Trigger	Coping strategy
Example	
Someone sitting next to me on the sofa	Tell myself the abuse is in the past and I am safe now. Try to relax. Write down my thoughts and feelings later

Trigger	Coping strategy
Example	

Examples

Trigger	Coping strategy
Maya	
Being presented with a plateful of food that my husband had cooked specially for me	Tell my husband it triggers off bad feelings. Say I don't want him to cook food specially for me. Write down feelings/flashbacks. Tolerate him sulking and feeling hurt without taking responsibility for it. Do something else, e.g. listen to relaxing music, exercise
Being on my own with a man, e.g. a patient at work	Explain to a colleague and work together where possible. Walk out of the room on pretext of getting records, equipment etc. Slow down breathing. Have a plan of what to do if he makes a sexual remark or tries to touch me, e.g. say, 'That is not what you are here for. You have come to have a medical so let's get on

Trigger	Coping strategy
	with it.' Refuse to continue if the bad behaviour continues. Call the police

Anthony

Passing the home of my abuser and the house where the abuse took place	Take a different route (avoid). Tell myself that the abuse is in the past and will not happen to me again

Jean

Smell a strong smell. (Sometimes I think this is the abuser coming to get me and it brings on a hallucination)	Check out where the smell is coming from. Tell myself, 'Don't let your imagination run away with itself'

Survivor's comment

This exercise helped me prepare and gave me a plan. I wrote out coping strategies and felt more positive and calmer and had clearer thoughts. I found the exercise empowering and it brought back memories of how healing it was to write. This is very positive stuff. MAYA

Dealing with flashbacks and hallucinations

Having a flashback or a hallucination is not necessarily a problem. The problem lies in the terror and powerlessness you experience because you believe you are a child again, that the abuse is happening again or the abuser is really present. To lessen this fear and help you feel more in control you need to try to stay in contact with the reality that you are an adult, that the abuser isn't really present and that you are re-experiencing things that happened in the past but aren't happening now. The aim at this stage is to help you overcome your fear of flashbacks and hallucinations, not necessarily to stop them. Below we discuss ways to help you do this.

Grounding exercises

Grounding exercises help to bring your focus back into the present.

- Focus on your breathing. Breathe slowly in through your nose and out through your mouth.
- Become aware of what is under your feet and your hands, e.g. the carpet under your feet, the wood of the chair arms under your hands.

- Make physical contact with an object associated with the present time. Keep an object with you that can act as a reminder that you are now an adult – choose an object that you did not have as a child. A ring, a bracelet, car keys or any object that will be easily accessible to you at all times is best.
- Hearing someone else's voice can help you to keep a link with the present time. If there is anyone with you ask them to keep talking to you – it doesn't matter what they say although reminding you where you are and how old you are is an added help.
- Follow the advice on reality orientation below.

EXERCISE 4.5   REALITY ORIENTATION

Reality orientation is about reminding yourself of your present situation as a way of understanding that you are no longer a child who is being abused. This helps to stop flashbacks and bring you back to your present reality. It can also help to use this after you have completed other exercises in this book or if you feel you are regressing to a child-like state.

Aim   To help you bring yourself back to present reality when you are about to have a flashback or you are in a flashback.

Get a small piece of card the size of a postcard and copy out sentences 1 to 6 below, filling in the blanks. If you live at the address where you were abused, miss out sentence 3. If you live with the person who abused you as a child or with any of the people you see in your flashbacks, miss out sentence 4. Keep this card with you at all times and if you are about to go into a flashback get it out and read it. Write down the answers again if you can.

1 My name is _____

2 I am _____ years old

3 I live at (write your address) _____

4 I live with _____

5 I work as _____

6 I have _____ children. They are called _____

Copy sentences 7–10 below and keep a copy with you at all times. Every time you are about to go into a flashback get this paper out and answer the following questions. Write the answers down if you can. Write down where you are and what you can see, hear and touch *in reality*. Don't write down the flashback.

7 I am in/at (where you are) _____

8 I can see _____

_____

_____

9 I can hear _____

_____

_____

10 I can touch _____

_____

_____

Example

1 My name is *Jenny Shaw*.
2 I am *37* years old.
3 I live at (write your address) *6, Westfield Rd, Wakefield*.
4 I live with *my partner and children*.
5 I work as *a part-time secretary*.
6 I have *2* children. They are called *Ben and Gillian*.
7 I am in/at *my living room*.
8 I can see *my TV, my settee, the photographs of my children, my potted plants*.
9 I can hear *the radio in the kitchen, the traffic outside*.
10 I can touch/feel *the carpet underneath my feet, the arms of the couch, the bracelet I bought two months ago*.

Dealing with flashbacks

Below are ten steps to help you deal with flashbacks. Photocopy this page or copy the steps out on to a piece of card and keep it with you at all times. When you feel a flashback coming on read the steps below and act on them. If there is someone you trust who would be willing to help you, prepare them in advance for what might happen by explaining to them about flashbacks. Ask them to help you work through these steps when you are having a flashback.

During the flashback

1 **Recognize and name what is happening.**
'I'm having a flashback.'
2 **Tell someone else what is happening.**
Even if you are not with people who know how to help you, it is worth

telling them that you need time and space to deal with what is happening to you.

3 **Remind yourself that the worst is over.**
E.g. 'This isn't happening now even if it feels as if it is. I'm remembering something that happened years ago. It's over.'

4 **Breathe slowly, focus on your breathing and ground yourself.**

5 **Re-orientate yourself to the present.**
Use Exercise 4.5 above.

6 **Remind yourself that you are an adult.**
Remind yourself that you are an adult now and try to calm and reassure the part of you that is frightened and feels as if you are a child.

After the flashback

7 **Take time to recover.**
Flashbacks can be emotionally and physically exhausting. Take time to recover – rest and be kind to yourself.

8 **Write down what happened in the flashback.**
The content of your flashback might provide useful information about what is still bothering you and what you are still having difficulty coming to terms with.

9 **Identify what triggered the flashback and write it down.**
Look back at Exercises 4.1 and 4.2.

10 **Learn from it.**
Although having a flashback can be very frightening it is not a sign of failure but an experience you can learn from and use. Could you have done anything differently?

Survivors' comments

I used to think flashbacks were my way of trying to punish myself. Now I realize it happens to other people. By writing your flashbacks down you can break the hold your abuser has on you. JEAN

1 Get your partner to ask you questions. Tell them not to be put off if you answer 'I don't know', or 'I can't remember'. It helps me if my partner says, 'I'll count to three slowly and then you tell me what is worrying you.'

2 Sometimes you might feel very anxious/depressed/agitated in the days or weeks prior to a particularly nasty memory coming up. Be aware of this.

3 Let yourself draw/write. Let the pen take over. Don't try and control your thoughts.

4 Keep a diary of dreams and flashbacks.
ANNABELLE

I was sick of being tortured by flashbacks and sick of harming myself. I am now learning to function as a competent adult, instead of being so helpless and out of control. MAYA

It is so frightening at the beginning, you feel that you are reliving the abuse all over again. You have to be strong and the flashbacks do get easier to deal with. I try to put my mind on to nice things rather than whatever is reminding me of the abuse. I also found that it helped me a lot to let a friend who understands talk to me. I am more in control of my flashbacks now. LESLEY-LEIGH

Dealing with hallucinations

We have worked with many Survivors who have suffered from hallucinations of their abusers. Over time they have managed to gain control of these experiences and eventually, by working on their past abuse, the hallucinations have stopped. Working on your feelings towards your abuser, overcoming fears about the consequences of speaking out, and realizing that your abuser no longer has power and control over your life is essential in this process. You will probably not be able to stop your hallucinations right now (in fact they could become more frequent as you work your way through this book), but there are techniques you can try to help lessen your fear and to gain some control over these experiences. We discuss these techniques below. Try them out and see what works for you.

- Throw something harmless like a screwed-up paper towel through the hallucination – Survivors are often amazed to find that the hallucination disappears. This can help to reduce your fears and increase your feelings of control and personal power. Always throw something light and harmless, not an object that could cause any damage. A paper towel works just as well as a hard object.

  I think the main thing is to be aware that although it seems real you can control it and you can be strong enough to say 'I'm going to stop this and get it into perspective'. If you are hallucinating build up some courage and go and touch the hallucination or throw something at it or shout at it. If you touch it and it disappears then you can see that it is not really there and you realize you are stronger and you have some control. YVONNE

- Reasoning can also help challenge the reality of hallucinations. Ask yourself how old the abuser looks and what he or she is wearing. In hallucinations abusers usually look the age they were when the abuse took place, maybe 10, 20 or 30 years previously, and are wearing the same clothes. By making these observations you will be able to reason with yourself – 'He looks like he's about 30 but he's actually in his mid 50s now so he can't be really here. I'm creating this image because of the fear in my mind.' Or, 'My abuser is dead so he cannot be here.'

- Remind yourself: 'This has happened before. I've seen my abuser and really believed she was with me but then realized that she couldn't have been.'
- Instead of keeping your experiences secret test their reality by sharing them with someone you trust and asking, 'Can you see/hear that too?'

Some Survivors have mixed feelings about trying to stop the hallucinations.

I feel safe in some ways when I have an hallucination because then I know where he is. I don't have to sit there and wonder when he will appear. JEAN

Think about whether you have any reasons for not wanting to stop the hallucinations.

Survivors' comments

The hallucinations are still with me but they are not as frequent and don't frighten me like they did at the onset. I have learnt how to deal with them. I tend to disregard them when they appear and carry on doing whatever I am doing. If they occur at night when it is dark and I see something which is odd I will turn the light on and have a look. The hallucination will not be present when I turn the light on. It somehow gives me a sort of power or to be more precise it gives me a sense of achievement. GRAHAM

I am no longer scared of my mother and I don't have the hallucinations anymore. GRAHAM (5 months later)

When my father [the abuser] first died and up until recently I really believed he was coming back from the dead to get at me. Now I'm beginning to think it's the fear in me that creates the image of him. I start thinking of all he said he could do. I imagine him being there and the fear is so intense that I see him and believe he really is there. I am now building up a resistance to this fear. JEAN

I used to smell my dad. He really had a strong hold on me. Now the hallucinations aren't as strong as they used to be. I see now that my mind conjured up an image of him that seemed so real. Now I accept that he can't come back to me. Because I'm now watching out for triggers it's making me think how to deal with them and to think of the positives. I have now got stronger and when I do see him I tell myself he is not real, it is my imagination. JEAN (2 months later)

Although it is possible to gain some control over your hallucinations by using these techniques and working through this book many Survivors will probably need to seek help from a therapist. Graham and Jean have both received therapy.

Make sure your therapist understands about trauma-based hallucinations and is willing to work with you on them. Not all therapists or mental health workers share this understanding of hallucinations, especially within psychiatry, and they may only be able to offer you medication. While medication can be helpful in alleviating symptoms it is rarely a long-term answer to the kind of hallucinations suffered by Survivors of sexual abuse that we have described here.

In section one of the book we have helped you look at how you have been affected by being abused and the strategies you use to try to cope, some of which may have become problems in their own right. The exercises in this chapter and the previous chapter help to prepare you for the work in the rest of the book. The previous chapter helped you to look at ways of coping with memories and feelings and to move towards using coping strategies that aren't going to cause you further problems. This chapter helped you to become aware of what triggers memories and feelings and to gain some control over these experiences. We hope that these exercises have helped you gain more understanding of your feelings and behaviours and helped prepare you for the work ahead. The next section of the book deals with guilt and self-blame.

II
Guilt and Self-Blame

Survivors often feel that they are responsible for being sexually abused. Many Survivors believe that they somehow caused the abuse to begin and that the abuse continued because they didn't stop it. Feeling guilty and blaming yourself for the abuse can undermine your self-confidence and prevent you from realizing your full potential.

Section II helps you to understand more about feelings of guilt and self-blame and to place the responsibility for abuse with the abuser.

In Chapter 5 you are asked to look at your beliefs that you are to blame because you didn't stop the abuse or tell anyone. Chapter 6 helps you to explore your beliefs that you may have caused the abuse to begin and helps you to understand more about how abuse is set up. Chapter 7 looks at why some Survivors find it difficult to let go of feelings of guilt and self-blame.

5
Why Didn't I Stop the Abuse?

This chapter begins by asking you to look at your current beliefs about who was responsible for the sexual abuse you experienced as a child. The rest of the chapter aims to help you challenge any thoughts that you were to blame because you didn't stop the abuse or tell anyone. Many Survivors have been abused by more than one person. If you have been abused by more than one person repeat the exercises in this chapter for each of your abusers. You can photocopy the exercises, write the exercises out again or use a different coloured pen for each abuser.

The next two exercises help you rate the extent to which you are currently blaming yourself for the abuse. Photocopy or make a written copy of Exercises 5.1 and 5.2 so that you can repeat them at the end of Chapter 8 and at other times whilst reading this book.

EXERCISE 5.1   RESPONSIBILITY CAKE
Aim   To see to what extent you think and feel that different people are responsible for the abuse you suffered.

It may help you complete this exercise if you first look at the example which follows.

Date _____

1   Who sexually abused you? _____
    (If you were abused by more than one person name one abuser each time you do the exercise.)
2   Write down all the people you think or feel might be responsible in any way for your abuse. _____

    _____

3 Below is a circle or 'cake'. Divide the cake into slices to represent how much you *think* each of the people above was responsible for the abuse you suffered.

How much I *think* each person was responsible for the abuse:

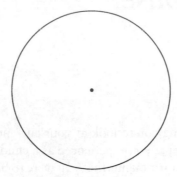

4 Now divide the cake below to show how much you *feel* each of the people above was responsible for your abuse.

How much I *feel* each person was responsible for the abuse:

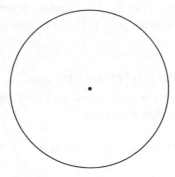

Note   You may find you divide the two cakes up in different ways. For example, some Survivors *know* (think) they are not responsible for the abuse but *feel* that they are partly responsible.

Rebecca's example

Below is an example of Rebecca's responsibility cakes. As we can see from the first circle Rebecca *thinks* her abuser is mostly responsible for the abuse but she also blames herself and her mother. However, when we look at the second circle we can see that she actually *feels* that she and her mother are more responsible for the abuse and feels her abuser has much less responsibility for what happened.

1   Who sexually abused you? ___*my dad*___

2   Write down all the people you think or feel might be responsible in any way for your abuse. ___*me, mother, the abuser*___

3   How much I *think* each person was responsible for the abuse:

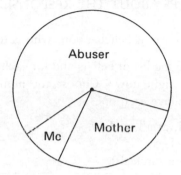

4   How much I *feel* each person was responsible for the abuse:

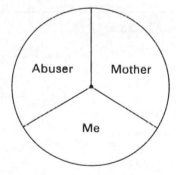

Survivor's comment

> While I was filling in the exercise I was constantly fighting the temptation to yet again accept all the responsibility for my abuse. It helped me to see the difference between what I think/know to be true and what I feel. They are very different things that are often confused. REBECCA

Beliefs about the responsibility for sexual abuse

We develop beliefs about ourselves in childhood as a result of our experiences and our interactions with other people and often hold these beliefs unchanged throughout our lives. For example, if you were brought up to believe that it didn't matter how you felt, you may grow up continuing to believe this is true. This exercise asks you to look at your beliefs about who is responsibility for sexual abuse and rate how strongly you believe them. Even though we may hold certain beliefs very strongly it does not mean they are true. The three chapters in this section help you to re-examine these beliefs as an adult to see how true they really are.

EXERCISE 5.2   BELIEFS ABOUT THE RESPONSIBILITY FOR SEXUAL ABUSE

Aim   To look at your current beliefs about who is to blame for the abuse.

Look through the following list of beliefs and for each one ask yourself: 'How much do I believe this right now?' Choose the number which corresponds with how much you believe each one:

- If you don't believe it at all circle 0.
- If you are unsure circle 5.
- If you totally believe it circle 10.

	Don't believe at all	?	Totally believe
I could not stop the abuse because the abuser had power over me	0 1 2 3 4 5 6 7 8 9 10		
There are good reasons why I couldn't tell anyone	0 1 2 3 4 5 6 7 8 9 10		
I was abused because an abuser had access to me not because of anything I had done	0 1 2 3 4 5 6 7 8 9 10		
Abusers are always responsible for abusing children	0 1 2 3 4 5 6 7 8 9 10		
I know my abuser was responsible for abusing me	0 1 2 3 4 5 6 7 8 9 10		
The abuse was definitely not my fault	0 1 2 3 4 5 6 7 8 9 1-0		
If you had more than one abuser:			
I had more than one abuser because several abusers had access to me	0 1 2 3 4 5 6 7 8 9 10		
I had more than one abuser because I was in a vulnerable and unprotected situation	0 1 2 3 4 5 6 7 8 9 10		

Why didn't I stop the abuse?

Sexual abuse is a trap. The abuser may use physical strength, power and authority, tricks, threats, treats or manipulation to coerce the child into the abuse and to keep them silent. Sexual abuse nearly always involves some form of relationship between the abuser and the child which is designed by the abuser to entrap the child and prevent him or her from stopping the abuse or telling anyone about it. Children are often sexually abused over weeks, months or many years, and often feel guilty because they believe they should have been able to stop the abuse or have told someone about it. They may believe that the abuse was at least partly their fault because they 'let' it go on for so long. For many Survivors the abuse continues after the age of 18 and may carry on into their twenties, thirties or later. This can add to the feelings of guilt and self-blame. Adults often carry the same beliefs and feelings of self-blame and shame they had as children and this can prevent them from talking about their abuse or seeking help to overcome their problems.

In the exercises below we help you to explore the reasons why you could not stop the abuse or tell anyone about it and to understand that you were not to blame for the abuse continuing over time.

Many of the following exercises ask you to think back to when you were a child. Use the ideas in Chapter 1 to keep safe and stay at the emotional distance from your past that allows you to think about what was happening without becoming too distressed. Repeat the exercises for each abuser if you have been abused by more than one person. When doing the exercises in this chapter, start with your first abuser because you will be looking at why you couldn't stop the abuse when it first started and how this makes it even more difficult for you to stop it later on.

The next three exercises explore the power that abusers have over their victims to help you see that children are not powerful enough to say 'No' or physically stop an abuser themselves.

Power

Adult Survivors often forget how powerless they were as children in comparison with their abusers. Abusers are often bigger than their victims, but physical size is only one type of power. They may be in a position of power because of their relationship or their role in the child's life, for example, parents have power over their children and school teachers have power over the children in their class. Abusers can also create a position of power over children by blackmailing them, threatening them or emotionally manipulating them. These sources of power can be more important than physical strength in controlling children. It is therefore possible for children to abuse other children of a similar size by exerting their power through emotional manipulation or through their position or role in their victims' lives. For example, an older sister may manipulate her siblings, a teenage babysitter has power over the children in his or her charge and a child may bully or abuse a classmate. Abusers misuse their power to frighten or control their victims.

EXERCISE 5.3 POWER

Aim To think about the kinds of power your abuser had over you to help you understand that you could not stop the abuse yourself.

1 What was the relationship of your abuser to yourself?

Abuser's name _____ Relationship to you _____
(For example, the relationship may be: parent, neighbour, priest, brother or sister, teacher, family friend, other child, stranger, babysitter.)

2 What kind of person was he or she?
(E.g. kind, well-respected, stern, bossy, violent, loving, feared.)

_____

_____

_____

_____

_____

3 Read through this list of the things that give abusers power over their victims and tick any that apply to you:

- You were told to obey adults.
- The abuser was an adult and you were a child.
- You wanted the abuser to love you so you wanted to please him or her.
- You loved the abuser and were scared of losing the relationship.
- The abuser was a bossy or bullying person and you were scared of him or her.
- The abuser was an older child.
- The abuser was ill or disabled and you felt sorry for him or her.
- The abuser was head of the family and told everyone what to do.
- The abuser was in a position of power over you (e.g. a teacher).
- The abuser was a respected person who was a powerful person in relation to adults as well (e.g. a priest).
- The abuser threatened or frightened you.
- The abuser was bigger and stronger than you.

Can you add any more?

-
-
-
-
-

> Adults are believed and children are thought to be the ones who tell lies.
> REBECCA

4 Write down the kinds of power or authority your abuser held over you. Think of your relationship with the abuser, his or her job, position in your community, and personality, and include any of the examples from above that apply to you.

_____

_____

_____

_____

_____

_____

_____

_____

_____

5 Do you know of anyone else your abuser had power over?
This does not have to be someone the abuser was *sexually* abusive to. It may even include animals or pets that the person was cruel to.
If so – who?

_____

_____

_____

_____

Survivor's comment

> Doing this exercise made me feel angry and sad as I realized how vulnerable I was. I told myself it is alright for me to feel this way. JEAN

I didn't say 'No'

> My mother was feared by everyone. She was a very strong member of the family who was always right. I never ever said 'NO' to her, I wouldn't dare. She knew I was scared of her. She never treated me as a child and she acted as if I was her property. GRAHAM

Many Survivors blame themselves for the abuse because, like Graham, they didn't say 'No' to their abusers. Graham was too scared of his mother to stand up to her or resist her. Other Survivors have been in a similar position because of the power their abusers held over them. To say 'No' to someone, you have to feel you have the power to do this and will be listened to. Children do not have this power in relation to their abusers. Even when children do say 'No', abusers often take no notice or may punish them for trying to resist.

Physical size of victims and abusers

When abuse begins, abusers are usually physically bigger and stronger than their victims. The following exercises aim to show you how difficult it would have been for you to stop an abuser who was bigger than you. The abuser may have been a similar size to you if the abuser was a child of a similar age or if you were a teenager when the abuse started. Remember, physical size is only one of the ways that abusers keep their victims trapped in abusive relationships.

EXERCISE 5.4   PHYSICAL SIZE OF VICTIMS AND ABUSERS
Aim   To look at the difference in physical size between children and adults.

1   How old were you when the abuse began? _____ years.
    Think about a child, *not yourself*, of this age (this could be a child you know or an imaginary child) or look at a child of this age.
    Compare the child's size and strength with that of an adult.

    Who is physically bigger or stronger? _____

    Would it be physically possible for the child to stop the adult from abusing him or her? Yes? No?

2 Draw a picture of a child (not yourself) of the same age you were when the abuse began.

Draw a picture of an adult. (Drawing stick people is fine.)

A child   **An adult**

Look at the difference in physical size.

Would it be physically possible for the child to stop the adult from abusing him or her? Yes? No?

3 Write down any thoughts or feelings that came up for you when you answered questions 1 and 2 above:

_____

_____

_____

_____

_____

Graham's example

 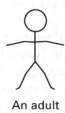

A child   An adult

EXERCISE 5.5   PHYSICAL SIZE OF YOU AND YOUR ABUSER

Aim   To help you see how difficult it would have been for you, as a child, to physically stop the abuser.

This exercise asks you to draw your abuser and yourself and look at photographs of your abuser and yourself as a child. If this feels too frightening for you, try using one of the distancing techniques from Chapter 1. For example, imagine you are looking at the photographs or drawings through the wrong end of a telescope to make them appear smaller and have a less powerful effect on you.

1   Draw a picture of yourself and the abuser at the time the abuse *began* – again stick drawings are fine. You may have been much older when the abuse ended but it is important that you draw yourself as you were at the time the abuse began.

This is me   **The abuser**

Compare the difference in size between yourself as a child and the abuser in the drawings.

Would it have been possible for you to physically stop the abuser from abusing you? Yes? No?

2   Find a photograph of yourself at the age the abuse *began*.

Compare the size of yourself in the photograph with an adult or, if possible, with a photograph of your abuser.

Would it be possible for you to physically stop the adult from abusing you? Yes? No?

3 Note here any thoughts or feelings that come up for you:

_____

_____

_____

_____

_____

_____

_____

Jean's example

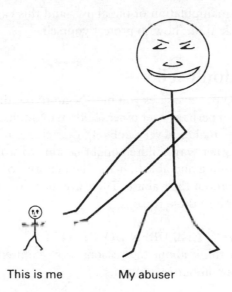

This is me   My abuser

Jean was so terrified of her abuser that she exaggerated his size in her drawing. He *was* much bigger than she was but her fear made him appear to her even bigger than he actually was.

Survivors' comments

I was a child. I was small. He was bigger than me. I was not strong enough to stop him. LESLEY-LEIGH

I felt terror, sadness, confusion, hatred and anger. I was sweating. I wanted to pick the child up and cuddle her, the child needed help. JEAN

Looking at the stick drawings of a child and an adult I can see the adult is at least three times bigger. When I draw myself and one of my abusers (my

mother) I can see she was bigger than me and a lot stronger but I should have
been able to stop the abuse when I was 15 and bigger than my mother.
GRAHAM

After doing this exercise you may, like Graham, be able to see that when the abuse
began you were too small to stop it but still think you should have been able to stop
the abuse when you were older and bigger. Male Survivors often feel especially
ashamed because they think they should have been physically strong enough to
stop their abusers, particularly when they became teenagers. Survivors, of either
sex, may think they should have been strong enough to stop abuse by women.
Remember that physical strength is only one form of power that abusers hold over
their victims. When abuse has gone on for some time you become trapped by the
emotional power and manipulation of the abuser and this can prevent you from
even beginning to think about how to protect yourself.

Why children don't tell

After completing the above exercises you may begin to see the ways your abuser
had power over you and perhaps over other children or adults. The power abusers
hold over their victims makes it very unlikely that children can stop the abuse
themselves. The only other way children might be able to stop abuse is to tell an
adult who would be willing and able to help. The majority of children do not feel
able to talk to anyone about their abuse. There are many reasons for this and the
following exercises explore these reasons.

EXERCISE 5.6 WHY CHILDREN DON'T TELL
Aim To help you think about the reasons why children and teenagers are
unable to tell anyone about sexual abuse.

If you have spent your life feeling ashamed and guilty about the abuse it may
be difficult to *think* about your own situation without being overwhelmed by
your feelings. When you do this exercise think about other children, of any
age, who are being sexually abused.

  There are many pressures on children to keep quiet about sexual abuse and
many reasons why they can't tell. Spend some time thinking about the reasons
why children can't tell anyone when they are being abused.

Thinking about the following things may help you do this exercise:

- What is the child afraid of?
- Why might it be difficult to talk about sexual things?
- What is the child feeling?
- What is the child's understanding of what is happening?

Write below any reasons you can think of why children can't tell:

-
-
-
-
-
-
-
-
-
-
-
-

EXERCISE 5.7   WHY CHILDREN CAN'T TELL

Aim   To increase your awareness of the reasons you could not tell about the abuse.

Below is a list of some of the reasons why children can't tell when they are being abused. Read through them and tick off any that applied to you. See if you can add any more.

Who to tell?	Applied to you?
Parents dead, ill, absent	
Parents involved in the abuse	
No trustworthy adult around	
No opportunity to talk alone with a trusted adult	
Care-givers do not listen	
Frightened of parents	
Parents discourage talk about sex	
No friends	
No one to tell	

What to say?

Too young to talk .... _____

Don't know how to describe what's happening .... _____

Too embarrassed and ashamed to say what is happening . _____

Fears about the consequences of telling

1 *Threats from the abuser*

No one will believe you .... _____

You will be put into a home/taken into care................. _____

You will not see your mother again .... _____

The family will be split up .... _____

Affection and love will be withdrawn........................ _____

Family and friends will reject you .... _____

No one will want to marry you .... _____

Threatened or actual physical violence to you, your family
 or pets .... _____

The abuser will commit suicide or be put in prison .... _____

2 *Fears about other people's reactions*

No one will believe you .... _____

Mother will feel guilty... _____

The family will be hurt.. _____

Mother/father will be upset...................................... _____

Mother will reject you .... _____

Other people will think you are to blame .... _____

Other people will think you are dirty, contaminated or
 disgusting.. _____

You will be rejected and the abuser supported .... _____

3 *Fears for the abuser*

The abuser will be hurt and rejected .... _____

The abuser will be put in prison .... _____

The abuser will get beaten up .... _____

The abuser will commit suicide .... _____

4 *Fears that telling won't help*

Nothing will change... _____

No one can stop it... _____

Events will get out of control.................................... _____

Fear of the unknown.. _____

Others seem to know anyway .... _____

It might get worse .... _____

The abuser is too powerful and can't be stopped .... _____

Applied to you?

The child's confusion

Feelings and thoughts which prevent children from telling include:

Feelings of guilt and self-blame................................ _____

Feelings of shame and embarrassment .... _____

Confusion – is it really happening? Is it wrong?........... _____

Thinking the abuse is normal.................................... _____

Not understanding what is happening .... _____

Believing you are the only one this has ever happened to.. _____

Feeling dirty, contaminated, polluted........................ _____

Feeling trapped by the secrecy................................ _____

Feeling you are being punished and deserve it.............. _____

Hoping the abuse won't happen again....................... _____

Blocking off all memories of the abuse .... _____

Feeling sorry for the abuser.................................... _____

Not wanting to betray the abuser by telling .... _____

Feeling it's your fault because you took sweets, money,
   toys or other rewards from the abuser .... _____

Enjoying the sexual stimulation .... _____

Enjoying the affection, warmth or closeness .... _____

Thinking 'I didn't tell when it first happened so how can
   I tell now?'... _____

Others:

_____ _____

_____ _____

_____ _____

_____ _____

_____ _____

_____ _____

_____ _____

There are many reasons why most children and young people who are being abused are unable to tell anyone about what is happening. Despite being under a lot of pressure to keep quiet at the time of the abuse, Survivors usually grow up blaming themselves for keeping the abuse secret. You have indicated on the list above the reasons why **you** were unable to tell and this may increase your awareness of the pressures that were on you to keep quiet. Survivors often find it helps them understand more about why they kept the secret to write their own account of why they couldn't tell.

EXERCISE 5.8   WHY *I* COULDN'T TELL

Aim   To help you understand the pressures that were on you to remain silent about the abuse.

Write an account of why you were unable to tell anyone about the abuse. Use your answers from the previous exercise to help you. If you don't want to write an account find some other way of representing why you couldn't tell, e.g. a cartoon strip or a spidergram (see Nina's example on the next page).

It might help to complete this exercise if you first try to answer the following questions.

- How old were you when the abuse first began?
- Who could you have told?
- How do you think other people would have reacted?
- What are the reasons why you couldn't tell someone straight away?
- What are the reasons why you couldn't tell when it had been happening for some time?

Why I couldn't tell

Examples

Nina

Nina and her sister spent their childhood in a local authority children's home. All the children in the home were sexually, physically and emotionally abused by the matron in charge of the home. This is why Nina didn't tell:

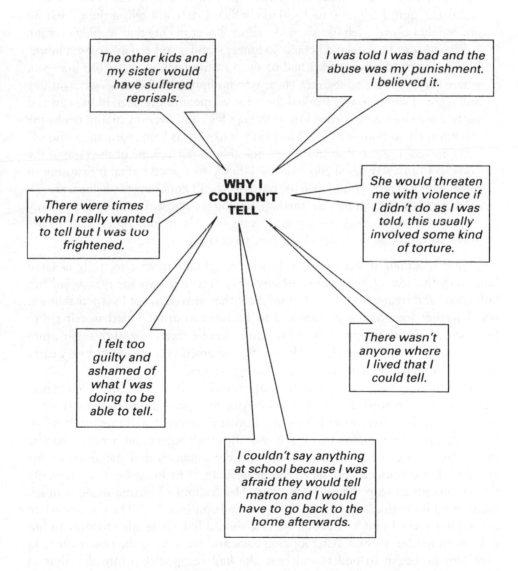

The other kids and my sister would have suffered reprisals.

I was told I was bad and the abuse was my punishment. I believed it.

WHY I COULDN'T TELL

There were times when I really wanted to tell but I was too frightened.

She would threaten me with violence if I didn't do as I was told, this usually involved some kind of torture.

I felt too guilty and ashamed of what I was doing to be able to tell.

There wasn't anyone where I lived that I could tell.

I couldn't say anything at school because I was afraid they would tell matron and I would have to go back to the home afterwards.

Jonathan

I loved my gran, she protected me from a very strict father. He could never understand why the grandmother of his five children chose to give *me* so much more in material things and love than she did the others. I was always being punished by my father or brothers and sisters who were jealous of the attention I was getting and said I was being spoiled by my gran. She started sexually abusing me when I was around three years old. She aroused me by hand and, as I got older, by mouth. When anybody told me how lucky I was to have such a wonderful gran I felt confused and in conflict. I dare not tell of things that no one would believe. I felt like she had a control over my life that would never go.

When I was 14 years old I could no longer stand it so I ran away from home. I got a job at a fairground. I had to sleep in the back of a big furniture van where they kept the generator. There was no light and the noise went on day and night. Two men who worked there forced me into the back of the van and pushed my face into a corner. One man kept his hand over my mouth whilst the other forced his body into me. The pain felt like I was being torn apart and my tears flowed. I felt so degraded I was not able to tell anyone of the rape of my body so I ran away again and went back home to a good hiding for causing so much worry. The rape and then the beating when I got home made me feel even more powerless. I couldn't do anything to stop the abuse. I could not reveal my secrets and so the abuse by my gran went on. My grandmother went to her grave with no one the wiser about her. JONATHAN

By giving Jonathan all her attention Jonathan's grandmother effectively isolated him from the rest of the family because they resented him for getting all her 'affection' and treats. It also made it unlikely that anyone would suspect that she was harming Jonathan who appeared to be her favourite. Jonathan felt guilty because he enjoyed the presents and the attention he received and this made him feel he was involved in the abuse. He also felt ashamed because, from a very early age, he responded sexually to her stimulating his penis.

Jonathan's unsuccessful attempt to escape the abuse by running away led to him feeling even more powerless to stop it. Looking at a photograph of himself when he was about five years old with his grandmother (Exercise 5.5) immediately made him realize that his grandmother was physically much bigger and stronger than he was at that time. However, he was still terribly ashamed that the abuse by his grandmother continued until he left home aged 18 as he knew he was physically strong enough to stop the abuse by then. His feelings of shame made it much harder for him to think about why the abuse had continued until he was in his late teens. He believed that as a young man he should have been able to stop an old woman from abusing him. After looking back and reassessing the power she held over him he began to understand how she had trapped him into the abusive relationship by confusing him and controlling his emotions. He became aware of her emotional power over him and how easy it was for her to manipulate him and the rest of his family. Jonathan's shame at his sexual response, his guilt at receiving all her attention and his feelings of total powerlessness left him feeling there was no way out. By looking back as an adult on his situation as a boy and a teenager and thinking about how he had been trapped Jonathan was at last able to break away from his shame and guilt and begin a new life.

Survivor's comment

> The exercise made me think carefully about the *real* reasons, not the imagined reasons, why I didn't tell. It was a relief to know I did have real reasons.
> REBECCA

Who would have listened?

Twenty years ago very few people were aware that so many children are sexually, physically and emotionally abused, and the majority of people would probably not have listened to or believed children who tried to disclose. If you had tried to disclose at that time you probably wouldn't have been protected. Over the last twenty years society's awareness of sexual abuse has gradually increased. Nowadays sexual abuse is talked about regularly on the television and radio and written about in newspapers and magazines. This increased awareness makes it more likely that children will be listened to and believed. However, there are still many people who would not listen to children or believe them and the pressures on children to keep the secret remain the same.

I did tell

In the past children who did tell often received a negative reaction or were not protected. You may have told someone who ignored you, didn't believe you, blamed you, was angry with you or did nothing to stop the abuse. These negative reactions could have made you feel you were not worth protecting or increased your feelings of shame and powerlessness. If you told and the abuse continued this may have increased your belief that the abuser could not be stopped and made it less likely that you would try to tell again. Children who disclose and receive negative reactions often retract and say the abuse didn't really happen.

People react to disclosures in negative ways for many reasons. Some find it hard to believe that sexual abuse happens, others have not dealt with their own childhood abuse or are frightened of the consequences of believing and supporting the Survivor. Their negative responses are due to problems within themselves not because you were not worth protecting. You should have been believed and protected. Chapter 9 explores why mothers or other caretakers don't always listen to children or protect them.

Children are not able to stop abuse themselves and are rarely able to tell anyone about what is happening. Understanding this can help you feel less responsible for the abuse but can also make you aware of how vulnerable and powerless you were as a child. In Chapter 7 we help you look at the power you have now as an adult. In the next chapter we continue to explore your beliefs that you are responsible for the abuse by looking at the reasons why children believe they somehow caused the abuse to begin.

6
Did I Cause the Abuse?

Survivors often believe that they caused the abuse to start or that they were specially chosen to be abused because of something about the way they were. These thoughts may not always be completely conscious but they can lead to deep feelings of guilt and shame. This chapter helps you to explore your beliefs about why the abuse began and to begin to see that the cause of the abuse lies within the abuser not with yourself.

If you have been abused by more than one person repeat the exercises in this chapter for each of your abusers, starting with the abuser that you feel easiest answering these questions about.

EXERCISE 6.1   DID I CAUSE THE ABUSE?
Aim   To help you become more aware of why you think you caused the abuse to begin.

Below is a list of reasons why Survivors sometimes think that they caused the abuse to happen or why they think they were specially chosen to be abused. For each of these reasons tick one of the four columns below. At the end of the list add any other reasons why you think you caused the abuse, or were chosen, and rate them in the same way.

	1 Doesn't apply to me	2 Definitely means I'm to blame	3 Could mean I'm to blame	4 Doesn't mean I'm to blame
I was:				
Flirtatious				
Naughty				
Well developed				
Bad				
Pretty				

89

	1 Doesn't apply to me	2 Definitely means I'm to blame	3 Could mean I'm to blame	4 Doesn't mean I'm to blame
I was:				
Ugly				
The oldest				
The youngest				
The middle one				
Quiet				
Lively				
Put on earth to be abused				
Too loving				
Not loving enough				
I showed my knickers				
I got in bed with the abuser				
I got into the bath with the abuser				
I cuddled the abuser				
I sat on the abuser's knee				
I gave out a sign to my abuser				
I enjoyed getting attention from the abuser				

Other reasons

Survivors' comments

> It did help me to identify those things I still had doubts about even after having had therapy. I kept on reminding myself that I knew I wasn't to blame even if I felt that I was. REBECCA

Jean filled this exercise in twice. The first time, she filled it in as she had been thinking as a child, showing that for many reasons she felt she was definitely to blame. The second time she filled it in as she is now, thinking as an adult, and indicated that she felt just a few of the reasons 'could mean I'm to blame'. She says:

> This exercise brought back memories I didn't want to remember. It took me a while to fill in. I kept putting the sheet down to get my composure back. Every time a bad memory came to me and I felt weepy I gave myself at least half an hour away from the exercise. JEAN

EXERCISE 6.2   WOULD YOU BLAME A CHILD?
Aim   To highlight any differences in the way you judge yourself and others.

Think of a child, maybe your own child, or a child of a friend or neighbour, or any child that you know or have seen. Imagine that the child tells about being sexually abused and says he or she caused it because of the reasons below. For each of the reasons that the child gives, tick one of the three columns to show how much you think that means the child is to blame for the abuse. Add your own reasons from the end of Exercise 6.1 and rate what you would think if the child gave you those reasons.

	The child is definitely to blame	The child could be to blame	The child isn't to blame
The child says he or she was:			
Flirtatious			
Naughty			
Well developed			
Bad			
Pretty			
Ugly			
The oldest			
The youngest			
The middle one			
Quiet			
Lively			

	The child is definitely to blame	The child could be to blame	The child isn't to blame
Fearful			
Put on earth to be abused	_____	_____	_____
Too loving	_____	_____	_____
Not loving enough	_____	_____	_____
The child says:			
I showed my knickers	_____	_____	_____
I got in bed with the abuser	_____	_____	_____
The child says:			
I got into the bath with the abuser	_____	_____	_____
I cuddled the abuser	_____	_____	_____
I sat on the abuser's knee	_____	_____	_____
I gave out a sign to my abuser	_____	_____	_____
I enjoyed getting attention from the abuser	_____	_____	_____
Other reasons			
_____	_____	_____	_____
_____	_____	_____	_____
_____	_____	_____	_____
_____	_____	_____	_____
_____	_____	_____	_____

When you have done this compare your answers to Exercise 6.1. Are you blaming yourself in ways you wouldn't blame this child? If so write down why this is below.

_____

_____

_____

_____

_____

_____

Survivors' comments

There is no way that I could imagine that an abused child could be apportioned blame of any kind. This exercise allowed me to put down on paper what I believed. I have given different answers to Exercises 6.1 and 6.2. I suppose this is because I still judge myself much harsher, not just with these questions but throughout day-to-day living. I expect a great deal more from myself than I do from others but I'm working on it! Try not to use your own situation when you do this exercise. ANITA

I had difficulty not getting me and the child mixed up. I wanted to fill the exercise in as if it were me. I was getting upset about it and angry because of where I had to put the ticks. My feelings about being abused came to the front and about how I thought about myself. I had to keep remembering that the child I was thinking about was not me. JEAN.

This is a very important exercise. It enabled me to see the way we develop double standards in dealing with ourselves and others. We are always ready to blame ourselves. I felt angry that I was often too eager to take the blame and responsibility for things I had no control over. I am probably blaming myself because these were some of the reasons given to me by my abusers and by some of the people I sought help from. They were also some of the reasons I invented for being abused. I needed reasons why I was treated like this. REBECCA

Finkelhor's model: Four steps before abuse occurs

In Chapter 2 we looked at Finkelhor's model about how abuse affects Survivors. David Finkelhor (1984) has also studied the situations in which sexual abuse occurs and found that four things must happen before a child is abused:

1 There is a person who wants to abuse.
2 The person overcomes thoughts that abusing is wrong.
3 The abuser gets the child alone.
4 The abuser overcomes the child's resistance.

Understanding more about this model can help Survivors challenge thoughts that they might have caused the abuse. You may feel angry or upset as you read more about the four steps below. Be prepared to have strong reactions and take a break when you need to.

1   There is a person who wants to abuse

For sexual abuse to occur there must first be a person who wants to abuse a child. Perhaps this sounds obvious but, as we have seen, many Survivors think the abuse started with themselves – their personality, appearance and behaviour. Abuse does not start with the child, abuse starts with the thoughts and desires of a person who wants to abuse children.

It is still not clear why certain people want to abuse children. There are no simple answers to this question but it is probable that there are a number of factors involved. What we do know is that a person doesn't come into contact with a certain child and suddenly becomes an abuser. Before the abuse occurs there is usually a period where the abuser fantasizes about what he or she is going to do to a child. The abuser's desire to abuse is not created by the child – it is there before the child appears.

In exercise 6.3 below is a list of factors that it is thought might contribute to a person wanting to abuse. They are not excuses or justifications for abuse and none of these factors in themselves explain why a person might abuse. For example, the majority of people who are abused as children *do not* go on to sexually abuse other people. Whatever the abuser's past experience, he or she is still responsible for the abuse. The problem lies within the abuser not within yourself.

EXERCISE 6.3   WHY YOUR ABUSER WANTED TO ABUSE

Aim   To help you understand that your abuser had a problem and was responsible for the abuse, not you.

Factors which might contribute to a person wanting to abuse

Tick off any of the following factors that you think might apply to your abuser.

Note   You are unlikely to know much about your abuser's motivation but you may be able to make guesses.

The abuser:	Applies to your abuser?
Was an authoritarian and controlling personality............	_____
Did not see children as other people but as objects to be used...	_____
Felt socially and sexually inadequate and insecure with other adults and wanted to abuse children to get sexual gratification without risk of rejection.......................	_____
Was sexually aroused by children.............................	_____
Was sexually, emotionally or physically abused as a child or adult and tried to make him or herself feel more powerful by victimizing someone else......................	_____
Was another child who was acting out things he or she had experienced or seen	_____

The abuser:	Applies to your abuser?
Felt powerless and wanted to exert control over children to feel more powerful	_____
Was full of anger and hate and a desire to hurt and control	_____

2 The person overcomes any thoughts that abusing is wrong

People who want to abuse know that it is wrong to abuse children. At the very least they know it is illegal. Before they can put their desires into action they have to deal with any thoughts they may have that abusing is wrong. Abusers may attempt to do this by **justifying** their behaviour, **normalizing** their behaviour or by **disinhibiting** themselves.

Justifying. Abusers manage to convince themselves that what they are doing is acceptable by justifying their behaviour to themselves in all sorts of ways. They may even justify their behaviour to the child they are abusing and convince the child that they have a good reason for abusing. Whatever an abuser thinks or says, there is no good reason for abuse. Abuse does not benefit the child.

Normalizing. Abusers can create environments for themselves where child sexual abuse is seen as acceptable or normal. The abuser may associate with other people who also abuse children, watch child pornography or read information and listen to comments that appear to support the abuse of children. Some paedophile groups, for example, argue that the age of consent should be abolished on the basis that they are concerned for the sexual rights of children. This can help potential abusers to convince themselves that having sex with children is a way of sexually liberating them.

Disinhibiting. Alcohol and drugs lower inhibitions and people may then do things that they already want to do but might not have dared to do when sober. Many abusers drink alcohol before abusing. Drinking alcohol or taking drugs does not cause a person to sexually abuse a child but if the person already wants to abuse it may release inhibitions and allow the abuser to act out his or her fantasies. Hypnosis, rituals and dissociation can also put people into altered states and disinhibit them.

EXERCISE 6.4   HOW YOUR ABUSER CAME TO BELIEVE THAT ABUSING WAS OK

Aim   To help you understand how abusers persuade themselves that it is OK to abuse and to see that your abuser is responsible for the abuse, not you.

Below is a list of some of the ways in which abusers overcome their knowledge that abuse is wrong in order to allow themselves to abuse. Tick off any that you think might apply to your abuser and add any others you can think of in the spaces below.

Note   Again you are unlikely to know the precise answer to this question but your abuser may have done or said things that give you a clue.

Justifications

(For ease of understanding, Survivors are referred to as 'she' in the section below. Abusers use the same justifications about boys.)

The abuser thinks or says:	Applies to your abuser?
I'm just loving her	____
It's not intercourse so it's not abuse	____
It's sex education	____
She's too young to remember anyway	____
I'm not hurting her	____
She enjoys it	____
The law doesn't understand the special relationship I have with my child	____
She's my stepdaughter not my real daughter so it doesn't count	____
She is very provocative	____
I was abused and it didn't harm me	____
She seduced me	____
She didn't say 'No'	____
	____
	____
	____

Normalize	Applies to your abuser?
Abused in groups with other abusers	____
Knew other abusers	____

Applies to
your abuser?

Read or watched child pornography .... _____

Member of paedophile group.................................. _____

Read information from paedophile groups.................. _____

Had sex with children in other countries where the age of
consent is lower or where there is a sex tourism
industry.. _____

_____ _____

_____ _____

_____ _____

_____ _____

Disinhibit themselves through:

Alcohol... _____

Drugs .... _____

Dissociation.. _____

Rituals.. _____

Other ways of entering altered states..................... _____

_____ _____

_____ _____

_____ _____

3   The abuser gets the child alone

For abuse to occur the abuser must get a child alone or at least away from adults
who would be protective. Many children may have come into contact with abusers
but have not been abused because the abuser did not get the opportunity. Children
who are abused are unlucky enough to have been alone with an abuser or away
from people who could protect them.

EXERCISE 6.5   HOW THE ABUSER GOT ACCESS TO YOU

Aim   To help you understand how your abuser got you on your own or away
from other people who might have protected you.

Below is a list of ways in which abusers manage to get children on their own
or away from people who would protect them. Tick off any of the ways that
your abuser used. Add any other methods that your abuser used at the end of
the list.

97

Applies to your abuser?

Baby-sitting/looking after me .... _____

Giving my mum money to go out .... _____

Getting friendly with my parent(s) .... _____

Taking me on trips .... _____

Asking me into his or her house to:

- do jobs .... _____
- give me sweets .... _____
- play .... _____
- see animals/toys etc. .... _____
- watch TV .... _____
- other .... _____

Offering me lifts .... _____

Coming into the bedroom at night .... _____

Sharing a bedroom with me .... _____

Bathing me .... _____

Putting me to bed .... _____

Helping me with my homework .... _____

Making me share a bed with him or her .... _____

Waiting until I got into bed with him or her .... _____

Frightening other people into not stopping the abuse ...... _____

Getting me into a shed/garage .... _____

Taking me to an allotment .... _____

Having a job which allowed access to children
    (e.g. teacher, social worker, priest) .... _____

Doing voluntary work which allowed access to children
    (e.g. youth club leader, scout/guide leader, Sunday
    school teacher) .... _____

Abusing me when other people were around without them
    seeing .... _____

Taking opportunities when:

- a parent was in hospital .... _____
- a parent was away from home .... _____

_____ _____

_____ _____

_____ _____

_____ _____

Applies to
your abuser?

_____   _____
_____   _____
_____   _____
_____   _____
_____   _____
_____   _____

Survivors' comments

> The exercise made me see how vulnerable I was. I allowed myself to cry. It made me think about where I stood and what part I played in it. I saw the situation and it hit me – I had nowhere to go. It happened in the bath, the bed, the corner. My dad [the abuser] was all around me and I couldn't get out. I'm beginning to see (not 100 per cent) that not all the abuse was my fault. I let them [parents] convince me that it was my fault. JEAN

> It was quite overwhelming to see on paper how easy it is for abusers to abuse and that with the right planning and manipulation children are at risk. REBECCA

> It made me see clearly that it was a plan and not some accident or chance. It helped me to stop making excuses for him [the abuser]. He thought about it and knew what he was doing. CATHERINE

4   The abuser overcomes the child's resistance

The child does not come into this situation until the end. The scene has already been set. A person who wants to abuse children has persuaded him- or herself that it is OK to abuse and has a way to get access to a child. The abuser only has to make sure he or she can overcome the child's resistance by manipulating or forcing the child into the abuse. It is very easy for abusers to do this.

EXERCISE 6.6   HOW THE ABUSER GOT YOU TO COMPLY
Aim   To help you understand how your abuser got you to go along with the abuse.

Below is a list of ways in which abusers get children to do what they want. Tick off any reasons that apply to you and add any others you can think of at the end of the list.

Applies to you?

Adult authority...   _____
Parental authority...   _____

Applies to you?

Authority of older child .... _____

Starting the abuse gradually .... _____

Starting the abuse when you were very young.............. _____

Telling you it was a secret .... _____

Making you feel sorry for him or her .... _____

Blaming you for the abuse .... _____

Threatening you... _____

Threatening others if you didn't comply.................... _____

Rewards... _____

Treats.. _____

Confusing you.. _____

The abuser was bigger than you .... _____

Violent to you.. _____

Violent to others.. _____

Giving you alcohol .... _____

Giving you drugs .... _____

Pretending it was a game...................................... _____

Threatening to abuse your brothers or sisters if you
    objected.. _____

_____ _____

_____ _____

_____ _____

_____ _____

_____ _____

_____ _____

These are some of the ways that abusers trick, trap and overpower children. You may have noticed that the ways abusers get children to do what they want are the same reasons that we discussed in the last chapter about why children don't stop the abuse or tell anyone. This is not a coincidence; it is in the abusers' interest to make sure that the child does not resist and remains silent about what is happening.

Jean's example

Jean ticked the following reasons: and added:

Adult authority   Said he was doing what fathers do

Parental authority   Said it was all right he was dad

Starting the abuse gradually   Said he loved me and it was OK

Telling me it was a secret
Made me feel sorry for him
Blamed me for what he was doing
Threatened me
Started the abuse when I was very young
Threats to others if I didn't comply
The abuser was bigger than me

Said it was loving him
He said I was his favourite

Catherine's example

I don't think he said anything directly but indirectly I felt there were threats to others if I didn't comply. Indirectly he let me know it made him happy. I could then see he was happy and not shouting at mum or hitting my brother.

Survivors' comments

I had feelings of being lost and alone and trapped when I was doing this exercise. Afterwards I took the dog for a walk. I felt I needed the open air atmosphere. It helped me think about the exercise again and what I had written. I always believed I could have stepped out of the bath or shouted out when I was in bed but fear was what kept me in there and my parents were the ones who put that fear in me. I am now finding the exercises easier to complete. I am beginning to realize that it was not all my fault. JEAN

It made me realize that children could not be blamed for any kind of abuse as they are innocent children. I know *I* was a child but I still think I could have somehow stopped the abuse. I am quite annoyed that I let my abusers get away with what they did. GRAHAM

I feel a little bit that my abuser wasn't consciously aware of the powerful effect he had just by being my dad, an adult etc. He couldn't appreciate how insignificant I felt in comparison. I can see how I was powerless. He was in total control and therefore totally to blame. CATHERINE

Why did the abuse happen to me?

A child does not cause abuse, an abuser does. For abuse to happen there must be a person who wants to abuse and who has overcome any misgivings they had about doing it. The abuser must then find a place and time when he or she can abuse undisturbed and frighten or persuade the child into complying. You were unlucky enough to have been in the wrong place at the wrong time.

Coral's example of Exercises 6.3–6.6

My abuser's motivation:
He wanted power and control.

How my abuser convinced himself it was OK to abuse:
He told himself (and me):
   This is what you want.
   It won't harm you.
   I'm showing you how much I love you.
   I'm widening your experience and teaching you about life.

How my abuser got access to me:
He homed in on my mother who was a single parent.
He took a special interest in her children.
He volunteered to look after us while my mother went out.
He took me down to his boat.

How my abuser got me to comply:
He told me it was a secret.
He told me that it was a game.
I was too young to understand it was wrong.
It started gradually so it had been going on a long time before I was aware
   something was wrong.
I was told by my mother to do what I was told by adults.
He threatened me.
He was physically violent to me.

By doing the last four exercises we hope you are now in a better position to see that your abuse was caused by your abuser not you. However, it is difficult suddenly to give up self-blaming thoughts and beliefs you have held for many years. The next two exercises help you to continue to challenge your thoughts and beliefs. Remember it will probably take longer to get over the feeling that you caused the abuse, but working on your thoughts is the first step.

EXERCISE 6.7   CHALLENGING THE CHILD'S SELF-BLAME
Go back to Exercise 6.1 and look at all the reasons you have put a tick against in either column 2 or 3. Write all these reasons down the left-hand side of this page under the example below. Now imagine that a child tells you he or she caused the abuse because of this reason. In the right-hand column write down how you would reply to make the child understand that this does not mean he or she is to blame.

Reason	Your reply
Example	
I cuddled him	Children like to be cuddled. He had no right to abuse you. You are not to blame

_____

_____

_____

_____

_____

_____

_____

_____

_____

_____

_____

_____

_____

Examples

Reason	Your reply
Jean	
I am the middle one	It is not your fault that you are in the middle. It doesn't give anyone any right to abuse you
I'm too loving	So you're too loving, so what? Again it is no excuse for abuse
I'm lively	You are just enjoying life
Graham	
I am the oldest	That does not mean you have to endure abuse by any one
I am too quiet	They abused your trust and your body – no one has this right
I was put on earth to be abused	No one is put on earth to be abused. It just seems this way when it is happening to you
Rebecca	
I am naughty	A naughty child needs discipline but does not deserve to be abused

Reason Lesley-Leigh	Your reply
I am well developed	He should have controlled himself. You are a child
I enjoyed it	It was a nice feeling but it was not your fault that he made you feel that way. He was responsible

Survivors' comments

I found it hard to challenge the child's reasons when I believed these were the reasons it was my fault. When you are a child you don't want to believe a parent is doing something bad so you try to find another explanation for being abused. It hurts me to realize these reasons aren't true. I've abused myself as well by putting a lot of blame on myself. It seems a weird thought that none of these reasons make it my fault. JEAN

I couldn't complete the replies to the child in this exercise for a week after filling the reasons in. I was angry that I was *still* stuck. Don't be surprised by your reactions. Work through it in your own time. You may have to re-visit it several times like I did. REBECCA

I thought of my children and what I would say to them if they said they had been abused. I know now that no matter what, a child is not to blame for the abuse. An adult should always get the blame. In most cases adults know what they are doing. They have to take responsibility for themselves. LESLEY-LEIGH

I felt a very powerful difference between me self-blaming and another child self-blaming. It seems bizarre we are so hard on ourselves but so keen to defend other victims of abuse. Until pointed out to us we can't see this. It helped to change my very fixed beliefs. CATHERINE

EXERCISE 6.8   WHAT JUSTIFIES ABUSE?

Aim   To help you understand that your abuser had no right to abuse you no matter what you were like or what you did or didn't do.

Put a tick in one of the three columns below.

	Definitely agree	Maybe agree	Do not agree
A child deserves to be abused if he or she does the following:			
Cuddles people			
Sits on someone's knee			

	Definitely agree	Maybe agree	Do not agree
Shows her knickers/ his underpants			
Walks around the house in night clothes			
Walks around the house in underwear			

A child deserves to be abused if he or she does the following:

Walks around the house with no clothes on			
Gets into bed with a parent			
Gets into bed with a relative			
Gets into bed with an adult			

A child deserves to be abused if he or she is the following:

Pretty/attractive			
Ugly			
Well developed			
Quiet			
Lively			
Shy			
Too loving			
Not loving			
Naughty			
Flirtatious			

Nothing justifies abuse. Children do not deserve to be abused no matter what they do or who they are. No matter what you were like, what you said or didn't say, what you did or didn't do, or how you were dressed, this did not cause you to be abused. You were abused because someone who wanted to abuse a child had access to you. Nothing you said or did could have altered the danger you were in. Even if you removed all your clothes and invited the adult to have sex with you, you are not to blame. It is the adult's responsibility not to sexually abuse a child.

Survivors' comments

> I was surprised that there were some things I wasn't so sure about. It is helpful to do this with someone you trust who you can talk to about it. REBECCA

> I had a lot of feelings of being a child. My mum said I mustn't walk around in nightclothes, I'd encourage him. She said, 'Don't let him see you in your nightie and he won't do anything.' I had to try to remember to do the exercise as a grown-up but my thoughts kept going back to being a child. As me now, as an adult, I would put them all under 'do not agree with this'. JEAN

> A child never deserves to be abused. CATHERINE

> Though I believe that the abuser is to blame I sometimes, even now, wonder if it was because I was too loving. Gladly, I now only give it a moment's thought when I feel a bit low. Having read back through the exercise I now know that it is not a child's fault whatever they do. As an adult you do know whether something is right or wrong in this kind of situation and for an adult to take advantage of a child is something I will never agree with or understand. ANITA

In this chapter we have looked at why you might feel you caused the abuse to happen and have tried to help you challenge these reasons. For abuse to occur a child has to be unlucky enough to be around a person who wants to abuse children and who has convinced him- or herself that it is OK to do so. It is then very easy for an abuser to get a child to comply. Nothing you did or said was the cause of your being sexually abused; adults are always responsible for sexually abusing a child. It can, however, be difficult suddenly to stop blaming yourself; this process can take some time. There are also specific reasons why it might be particularly difficult to let go of guilt and self-blame. These are explored in the next chapter.

7
But I Still Feel Guilty...

Survivors often struggle to let go of their feelings of guilt. After working through Chapters 5 and 6 you may still feel guilty and believe the abuse was your fault. In this chapter we look at some of the things that can make it particularly difficult for Survivors to let go of guilt and help you explore why *you* may still feel to blame.

EXERCISE 7.1   WHY DO I STILL FEEL GUILTY?
Aim   To help you explore why you might find it difficult to let go of guilt.

Below are some of the thoughts and feelings that prevent Survivors letting go of their guilt. Some of them may be reasons that Survivors are aware of, whilst others may be underlying thoughts and feelings which they are not consciously aware of. Read through the list of reasons and see if any relate to you.

1 **I got something out of it.**
   You may think you were involved in the abuse or wanted the abuse because you got something out of it like attention, money or sexual pleasure.
2 **I had more than one abuser.**
   If you had several abusers you may believe you must have somehow drawn or attracted the abusers to yourself.
3 **I was the only person my abuser abused.**
   Thinking you were the only victim of your abuser can make you believe you were specially chosen.
4 **I'm frightened of feeling powerless.**
   Believing there was nothing you could do to stop the abuse can be very threatening because it leaves you feeling you had no control over what happened. To avoid feeling powerless in this way Survivors sometimes hold on to the idea that they must have caused the abuse or there must have been something they could have done to stop it.
5 **I don't want to damage my relationship with the abuser.**
   Survivors are sometimes afraid of believing their abusers are responsible for the abuse because they do not want to damage or lose their relationship

with the abuser. It can sometimes seem better to continue believing you were responsible for the abuse in order to maintain your relationship with the abuser.

6 **I'm frightened of my anger.**

Sometimes Survivors are afraid that if they accept that their abusers are responsible for the abuse they will not be able to contain their feelings of anger and will lose control of their behaviour.

7 **I know it wasn't my fault but I still *feel* guilty.**

You may know logically or objectively that it could not have been your fault but you still feel guilty.

Write here any of the above which might apply to you and any other reasons why you still feel to blame for the abuse:

_____

_____

_____

_____

_____

_____

_____

The reasons above can make it difficult for you to accept that you are not to blame for the abuse. The suggestions and exercises in the rest of this chapter help you explore and challenge each of these reasons.

Examples

I have been abused by so many people that I have always believed that I must have wanted it to happen and that I must have caused so many people to abuse me. After all *I* was the one they were all drawn to. SARAH

I know in reality I was not big enough or powerful enough to stop the abuse but I still think there must have been something that I could have done to stop it. I could and should have stopped it. GRAHAM

1   I got something out of it

I loved my family despite the abuse and I knew they wanted me to do well at school. I feel guilty because when a teacher began abusing me as well I sought him out in the hope of getting good marks to please my family and to give myself a future. THOMAS

Survivors often feel guilty because they enjoyed some aspect of the abuse or felt they got something out of it. Like Thomas, they may have sought their abusers out because there was something they wanted from them.

In Chapter 5 we saw how abusers have many different ways of getting children to go along with the abuse. They may use threats but they often offer children something that the children want or need in order to form a relationship with them and keep them involved in the abuse. For instance, a child who is neglected at home may be given much-wanted attention and this makes the child want to spend time with the abuser. Later this makes it difficult for the child to tell anyone because the child believes he or she encouraged the abuse by seeking out or accepting attention. This is part of the abuser's plan.

You may have got something you wanted from your relationship with the abuser, such as attention, gifts or cuddles. Receiving these things or seeking out the abuser for these things does not mean you wanted to be abused – it means the abuser was offering you things you wanted so you would be available for abuse.

EXERCISE 7.2 I GOT SOMETHING OUT OF IT
Aim To show you that you are not responsible for the abuse if you got something out of it.

Look at the list below and tick any that applied to you and add anything else you got from the abuse at the end:

	Applied to you?
I wanted the attention	
I wanted the affection.	
I liked being special	
I liked the presents/money.	
I enjoyed being taken out by the abuser	
I wanted to keep my relationship with the abuser	
I wanted the abuser to protect me from others	
I enjoyed the sexual arousal	
I wanted to be cuddled	
I wanted other things that I got out of it:	

109

Do you know why you wanted these things?

Sarah's example

> I wanted attention and kindness from my abusers.
>
> I wanted this because I was emotionally neglected by my family and craved attention from anyone – although I usually got the wrong kind of attention. I looked neglected and vulnerable. The abusers were often kind to me to start with so I enjoyed the attention. This made me believe I must have wanted the abuse.

Jonathan's story of why he didn't tell (example of Exercise 5.8) illustrates how knowing you got something from the abusive relationship can make you feel involved in the abuse or responsible for it. Jonathan enjoyed the attention and presents he received from his grandmother and he responded sexually to her stimulation of his penis. He felt very ashamed of his sexual response and this made it much more difficult for him to tell anyone or escape from the abuse.

Many Survivors become sexually aroused during their childhood abuse. They may enjoy the physical sensations, or have orgasms, and boys may show visible signs of arousal such as having an erection or ejaculating. Your sexual organs are designed to respond to sexual stimulation, so responding sexually is a sign that your body is working as it is supposed to. Boys can have erections as a reflex response to stimulation of their genitals or anal penetration. If you enjoyed the sexual feelings or sought them out it does not mean you were to blame for the abuse. The abuser used your sexual response to keep you in the abusive relationship. Your sexual feelings may have confused you or made you feel too involved or too ashamed to tell anyone.

As teenagers Survivors may realize more fully that the abuse is not right but continue to submit to it or even seek out the abuser in order to obtain money or other things that they want. This can add to their feelings of guilt and can be very difficult to come to terms with. If this happened to you it is important to remember how this situation came about – you were taught by the abuser that sexual behaviour could be exchanged for other things. This is a dangerous and confusing message for a child or teenager to receive and your abuser is responsible for teaching you to think and behave in this way. It is not surprising you tried to get what you could from an abusive situation.

The abuse was the responsibility of the abuser even if you gained something from it. The abuser used your wants and needs to manipulate you and commit a crime against you – you were not to blame.

2   I had more than one abuser

When you have been abused by two or more people it is easy to think that *you* were the common factor and that somehow you drew the abusers to yourself or it must have been something about you that caused it to happen.

> I was abused by lots of people because I am not the same as everybody else and something about me seems to make me get abused. There was some kind of attraction to me. GRAHAM

It is not unusual for Survivors to have been abused by more than one person; more than half of the Survivors we have worked with had several abusers. Some Survivors have said they felt they had a sign on their foreheads inviting people to abuse them. The next exercise aims to help Survivors who have had more than one abuser think again about why this might have happened.

EXERCISE 7.3   MULTIPLE ABUSERS
Aim   To help you understand why an abused child may be vulnerable to further abuse by other people.

This exercise is for people who have been abused (as a child or adult) by more than one person.
Note   For ease of understanding the victim is referred to as 'she' in the list below.

A   Think about a child who has already been sexually abused. Read this list of reasons why she or he may be vulnerable to being abused again by someone else and tick the columns on the right according to whether you think this reason:

Would make the child vulnerable to further abuse = **Yes**
Might make the child vulnerable to further abuse = **?**
Would not make the child vulnerable to further abuse = **No**

Reasons why a child who has already been sexually abused might be vulnerable to further abuse:	Makes the child vulnerable to further abuse?		
	Yes	?	No
She has no adult who will listen to her or believe her	_____	_____	_____
One or both of her parents has already abused her so she has no one to tell	_____	_____	_____

Reasons why a child who has already been sexually abused might be vulnerable to further abuse:	Makes the child vulnerable to further abuse?		
	Yes	?	No
She has no parents			
Her parents are unwilling to protect her			
Her parents encourage other people to abuse her			
The abuser passes the child or the child's name on to others			
Her mother has lots of boyfriends			
Her parents take in lodgers so many people have access to her			
She couldn't stop the abuse the first time so she doesn't believe she can the next time			
She can be blackmailed by someone who knows about the earlier abuse			
She blames herself for the first abuse and thinks she deserves any further abuse			
It's all she has ever known			
She thinks that abuse is all she is good for			

Add any other reasons you can think of below:

Survivors who have been abused by more than one person often feel that this proves that it must be something about them which caused this to happen. However, they were vulnerable to further abuse because of the situation they were in. In Chapter 6 we looked at Finkelhor's model which describes the four steps which must occur before a child is abused. Steps 3 and 4 in this model help us understand why it is common for a child to be abused by more than one person.

Step 3: The abuser gets the child alone. Children are vulnerable to abuse by several people if they are in a situation which makes it easy for abusers to get access to them. This can happen when, for example, a family takes in lodgers or uses many different babysitters or if the child lives away from home in local authority

112

care or at boarding school. The danger of further abuse is also increased if children have no one to protect them, for example when a child has abusive or neglectful parents, no parents or parents who are regularly absent or ill.

Step 4: The abuser overcomes the child's resistance. Sexual abuse often results in children feeling powerless and unable to protect themselves. It is easy for another abuser to control a child who has already learnt to do as she or he is told and remain silent. Some children feel so helpless and have been abused so often that they begin to accept abuse as inevitable and as a 'normal' situation which has to be tolerated.

> **Children are only abused by more than one abuser because they are unprotected and several abusers have access to them – not because of who they are.**

Adult Survivors may also be vulnerable to further abuse because they feel powerless and unable to defend themselves, they think abuse is 'normal', they believe they deserve to be abused and they may have had little experience of non-abusive relationships.

B Think about your own situation and write down why you think *you* were abused by more than one person. You may want to write an account of your own experience or write a list of reasons. Use the list above to give you some ideas.

When I was doing this exercise it helped me to think of a child I know being in the same situation that I was in and to imagine what she felt. SARAH

Why I was abused by more than one person

_____

_____

_____

_____

_____

_____

_____

_____

_____

Examples

Pauline

I thought it was my fault that I was abused by so many people because they could sense that I would let them. Doing this exercise made me realize that I couldn't have done anything at the time. I can see and understand how things were for me then. I was too frightened to say 'No' and it felt like everybody knew that I would let them do whatever they wanted. They knew I was vulnerable and they could get away with it because I daren't say anything to anybody. I feared for my life. I'd been abused by so many people I thought that everyone must have known what was happening. It felt like I deserved to be abused and I thought they might love me if I let them do it.

Now I know that I was abused by so many people because there were so many abusers around me and each one of the pathetic beings had access to *ME*.

Sarah

I was exposed to abuse from a very early age so I never learnt that I had a right to say 'No'. It was all I ever knew.

My parents took in lodgers and several of them abused me. I recently discovered that one of the lodgers had been accused of molesting little girls.

My name was passed round from one abuser to another.

Survivor's comments

Sarah felt distressed and angry after she had done the exercise. This is how she coped with her feelings.

I cried a lot. I dealt with my anger by punching my punch-bag. I then found it really helped to write letters (for myself – not to send) to all my abusers telling them how I felt and how pathetic they were.

Although the exercise brought up strong feelings Sarah found it very useful.

I have been abused by so many people that I have always believed that I must have wanted it to happen and that *I* must have caused so many people to abuse me. After all I was the one they were all drawn to. I felt relief when I did this exercise because I began to recognize that I did not want the abuse or cause it. I also felt angry that the abusers were so weak that they had to prey on a helpless, vulnerable child. It feels like the beginning of letting go of the guilt and responsibility.

3   I was the only person my abuser abused

Sometimes abusers do just abuse one child in a family. They often find ways of isolating the child from the rest of the family by making him or her feel different or special, as in Jonathan's situation where his grandmother singled him out for treats and special attention. Abusers may tell their victims they chose them because they were special, because they loved them, because they were bad and they were punishing them or for any of the other reasons described in Chapter 6. They find ways of making their victims feel responsible for the abuse in order to manipulate them into keeping silent. Even if you were the only victim, your abuser is still responsible for the abuse.

However, most abusers do not usually select one 'special' child to abuse and then stop. They go on abusing children whenever they get the opportunity or can create an opportunity. Abusers often have many victims who may be from inside or outside the family. Sisters and brothers may each spend years believing they are the only one in the family who has been abused. If one person has been keeping the abuse secret other people have probably been doing the same thing. You may think you were the only child chosen by your abuser when in reality he or she abused several other children as well. Survivors frequently discover, as adults, that family members or other people have also been abused by the same person.

4   Powerlessness

Doing the exercises in Chapter 5 made me see that my abusers were at least twice as big as me and over twenty years older. I felt overwhelmed, small and insignificant. I feel angry with the abusers because I was so little and weak and unable to protect myself. I got angry about the power imbalance between me and them. Although it helped me see how I couldn't stop the abuse it left me feeling powerless and vulnerable. REBECCA

When you believe you are to blame for the abuse you can at least feel you had some control over what was happening. Realizing you did not cause the abuse and could not stop it can relieve feelings of guilt but it can also be very frightening to realize you had no control over the situation and were so powerless. Feeling powerless or your fear of being powerless can make it difficult to let go of feelings of self-blame.

I coped with feeling so powerless and vulnerable by talking it through with someone and reminding myself that things are different now and I am no longer that child. REBECCA

You *were* powerless and vulnerable as a child but you are an adult now. The next two exercises are designed to help you become more aware of the greater strength and power you have now.

Your physical size and power now

Exercise 5.4 looked at how your abuser was probably bigger and stronger than you were when the abuse began, to help you see you could not have physically stopped the abuser. In the next exercise you are asked to compare the size you are now with your abuser's current size. It is important that you draw your abuser at the actual size he or she is now, not how big you *feel* he or she is. When we are frightened of someone we sometimes imagine that they are bigger than they actually are. Try to distance yourself from your feelings about the abuser if you can and think objectively about what he or her actual size is now.

EXERCISE 7.5   PHYSICAL SIZE NOW

Aim   To help you feel less powerless in relation to your abuser by looking at the difference in physical size between you and your abuser now.

Draw a picture of yourself and your abuser as you both are now. (Drawing stick figures is fine.)

                    Me as I am now   My abuser now

There is probably much less difference in size between you and the abuser now compared to when the abuse began. Some of you will now be bigger than your abuser.

Write down any thoughts and feelings that came up for you when you were doing this exercise:

_____

_____

_____

_____

_____

_____

_____

Survivor's comment

> I'm the same size as my mother now and I realize it can never happen again.
> GRAHAM

You may be feeling vulnerable because your abuser is still bigger than you or because it still feels like the abuser has all the power. The next exercise helps you look at the difference between the power you had at the time of the abuse and the power you have now. It is useful to do this exercise even if your abuse is ongoing.

EXERCISE 7.6   POWER NOW

Aim   To help you see the abuser no longer holds all the power by looking at the power you have now.

In Exercise 5.3 you looked at the kinds of power your abuser had over you as a child. You do have more power now than you did then even though you may not be aware of it. In this exercise you will be looking at the kinds of power you have now. Below is a list of some of the reasons why children are powerless *at the time of the abuse* and also why adult Survivors *do* have more power *now*. Read the list and tick off any of the statements that apply to you. Add any more reasons why you have more power now.

During the abuse you were:	Applies to you?	Now you are:	Applies to you?
A child or teenager	_____	An adult	_____
Physically small	_____	Physically larger	_____
Trapped by the abuser	_____	Not trapped by the abuser	_____
Powerless	_____	Working on taking control	_____
Silenced by the secret	_____	Telling or thinking of telling someone	_____
Dependent on the abuser	_____	Not dependent on the abuser	_____

During the abuse you had:		Now you have:	
No knowledge of abuse	_____	Information and knowledge	_____
No one around who would have believed you	_____	People around who know and believe about child abuse	_____
No one to tell	_____	People you could tell	_____

During the abuse:	Applies to you?	Now:	Applies to you?
The abuser was strong	_____	The abuser is older, weaker or dead	_____
You were confused about what was happening	_____	You know it was abuse and it was illegal	_____
You blamed yourself	_____	You know the abuser was responsible	_____
_____	_____	_____	_____
_____	_____	_____	_____

Write down any sources of power you have now that you did not have as a child. (Use the list above to help you.)

_____

_____

_____

_____

_____

_____

_____

Although Survivors often feel powerless they have much more power as an adult than they did as children. The exercise above may have increased your awareness of the power you have now. By working through this book you are gradually building up your own power and strength.

Survivor's comment

I realized I can get out of my abuser's clutch – it is coming. I am getting there, I am stronger now. JEAN

It's a crime

As a child I was powerless and I was blackmailed not to tell anyone. Now I've had therapy I have been confident enough to tell the police and the courts. This helped me get my power back. PAULINE

Having any form of sexual contact with a child is *a crime* even if the child 'agreed' to it. One form of power you have now is the knowledge that the abuser committed

118

a crime and that you have the power to report the abuser to the police. We are not suggesting that you do go to the police. This is something that needs to be thought about carefully and you need to be prepared for what might happen. There are no time limits on prosecution for major crimes such as child abuse but there is rarely enough evidence to successfully prosecute for abuse that happened years ago. What is important is that you are aware that the abuser committed an illegal act and that you know you have the power to inform the police and that they would take your report seriously.

> *Note* If you do decide to report your abuser to the police it is important to talk it through with someone first so you are fully aware of the consequences and how you may be affected. Contact one of the phone-lines in the sources of help section at the end of the book.

As a child you were under the power of your abuser. You may have learnt to initiate the abuse or seek out the abuser so you could at least feel you had some control over what was happening. This may have helped you survive the abuse instead of feeling totally powerless. As an adult you may still feel to blame for the abuse because you feel you should have been able to stop it or because you sought the abuser out. It may be difficult to give up feeling responsible for the abuse because you are afraid you will then feel totally powerless. To overcome this you need to accept that you were powerless as a child and therefore not responsible for the abuse but that you are not powerless now. Your power is growing as you release the guilt that is holding you back and as you break free from the effects of the abuse.

You may still have symptoms that make you feel out of control such as panic attacks and sleep problems, and you may be using coping strategies such as obsessional-compulsive behaviours, being aggressive, and controlling your body size and eating to make you feel more in control of your life. If you feel out of control or experience any of these problems remind yourself you have greater strength and power now than you did as a child. Learning to take control of your symptoms will help you feel more powerful and more in control of your life and this may also enable you to release the feelings of guilt. Some of these problems can be difficult to overcome by yourself and you may need to seek professional help.

5   Relationship with the abuser

Survivors are often afraid of placing the responsibility for the abuse with their abusers because they do not want to damage their relationship with the abuser or change their view of him or her. Children are dependent on their families or care-givers for their emotional and physical well-being and usually want to keep their relationships with them even if these are the people who are abusing them. Adult Survivors may feel loyal to their abusers, especially if they are family members, and feel they would be betraying them if they blame them for the abuse. However, it is abusers who betray the trust of children in their care and they are responsible for their actions.

All children want to feel loved by their parents and other people close to them. Being abused by a parent or someone you love can create a huge inner conflict. It is hard to believe that someone who loves you could deliberately harm you. Sometimes children find it easier to believe the abuse was their fault rather than face up to the fact that the abuser was willing to harm them for his or her own desires. Survivors may believe they somehow caused the abuser to abuse them and they sometimes say things like 'It was my fault because I was naughty', or 'He only did it because I wanted him to'. By taking on the responsibility for the abuse, the Survivor can continue to see the abuser as a loving, caring person.

Annabelle loved her father and found it hard to accept he had abused her. As a child she had separated him in her mind into two people – a loving father and the 'bye-bye man' who abused her in the night:

> It would be much easier to come to terms with having been abused if your abuser was an ugly stranger. When that person is your father, someone you would expect to love and protect you, then it all becomes more complicated. To see your father as one who is capable of terrifying his own child into participating in sexual activities is so devastatingly threatening that you prefer to doubt your own experience and sanity. You need a father who is kind and protective, not the 'bye-bye man' who lurks in the shadow of your bedroom. You become very protective towards your abuser and start to idealize him. Whatever he says or does is always right. You feel special when you are with him and want that to continue. You seek out sexual activity and you may actually enjoy what is happening and experience orgasms. You cannot let your mother know as you have been a willing part of it. She would accuse you of being wicked and a slut and she would be right. ANNABELLE

Annabelle could not see her father as responsible for the abuse because she wanted to retain her memories of a loving relationship with him. She saw her father as someone who never did anything wrong and instead blamed herself for seeking him out for attention and sexual activity.

Think about the following questions:

- Were you emotionally or physically dependent on your abuser?
- Was the relationship with the abuser important to you?
- Do you love your abuser?

If you answered 'Yes' to any of these questions and you are still blaming yourself for the abuse you may be trying to protect your abuser or your relationship with your abuser. Try to accept that you may have tolerated the sexual acts or sought out the abuser because you wanted to keep your relationship with the abuser or your view of the abuser as a caring person. The sexual activity was the responsibility of the abuser – you were not to blame. You do not have to continue holding yourself responsible for the abuse in order to maintain your relationship with the abuser. It is possible to carry on loving someone as well as giving him or her the responsibility for the abuse.

6 Anger

Once you begin to realize that you are not to blame for the abuse you may start to feel very angry. Some Survivors describe how their feelings of rage and hatred are so powerful that they fear they will not be able to contain them. They may fear they will act inappropriately or become aggressive or violent. Survivors describe urges to go out and confront their abusers or attack them or even kill them. Angry feelings may also be directed at other people, such as the non-abusing parent who failed to protect, or at people who do not understand. Some Survivors have learnt to turn their anger on themselves and may fear they will harm themselves.

Angry feelings like this can be very frightening and overwhelming and it is no wonder that some Survivors retreat back into blaming themselves for the abuse. Blaming yourself can be easier and more comfortable than dealing with feelings of murderous rage. Survivors have usually been unable to express their anger directly during their childhood and so have had to find other ways of dealing with it. Blaming yourself can also be seen as a coping strategy – a way of containing your anger and keeping yourself and other people safe. It is not always easy to know whether you are blaming yourself as a way of containing your anger. Many of these processes happen outside our conscious awareness. Try to answer the questions below without censoring your thoughts and feelings.

- **If you stop blaming yourself for the abuse who or what might you feel angry with?**

_____

_____

_____

_____

_____

_____

_____

121

- What do you fear you might do or what might happen if you experienced that anger?

_____

_____

_____

_____

_____

Here are a few suggestions:

- Accept that your guilt may be a way of containing your anger. When you feel more confident about dealing with your anger safely you will be in a better position to let go of the guilt.
- Work on being assertive, and acknowledging and dealing with feelings of anger in everyday situations as they arise rather than bottling up your anger.
- Remember that having feelings of anger and thoughts of revenge is a common reaction to trauma. Many people experience these thoughts and feelings but do not act on them.
- If you feel tempted to act violently, think about the consequences. Violence can feel like a solution but actually creates more problems.
- If you think there is a serious danger that you will actually harm someone else or yourself, seek professional help.
- Anger can be expressed safely and non-violently. Explore ways of dealing with your anger by reading a book about it, talking to other people about how they cope, or working with a therapist. The next exercise will help you find ways of coping with your anger.

EXERCISE 7.7   SAFE WAYS OF EXPRESSING ANGER
Aim   To help you find ways of expressing your anger safely and non-violently.

Write a list below of all the ways you could express your anger safely and without harming yourself or others. It may help to ask other people how they cope with anger.

_____

_____

_____

_____

_____

Example

This is a list produced by a Wakefield Survivors' group:

Shout	Write a letter
Phone someone	Punch my punchbag
Write down how I feel	Talk into a tape
Paint or draw	Hit a cushion/hit the bed
Talk to a chair	Use a stress doll
Talk to a counsellor	Do physical exercise

7   I know it wasn't my fault but I still *feel* guilty

You may now understand that you couldn't stop the abuse or tell anyone and that it was *not* your fault that you were abused or that the abuse continued over months or years. However, you may still *feel* it was your fault. It is easier to change the way you think than to change the way you feel. It often takes time for changes in your feelings to catch up with changes in the way you think. Whenever you feel guilty look through the last two chapters again. Better still – *do* the exercises again. Over time this will help your feelings change as well as your beliefs so you no longer *feel* you are to blame or *feel* guilty. Try the next exercise.

EXERCISE 7.8   ABUSERS ARE ALWAYS RESPONSIBLE FOR ABUSE

Aim   To remind yourself every day that you are not responsible for the abuse.

It takes time to change feelings you have had for many years but regularly challenging your old beliefs can help this change to occur. Write the following words on a piece of paper and put the paper somewhere where you will see the words every day or say them to yourself every morning.

> It doesn't matter what a child does. Sexual abuse only occurs when an abuser has access to a child. Abusers are *always* responsible for abuse.

> It doesn't matter what I did. I was sexually abused because an abuser had access to me.

Guilt, shame and blame

Why not try Exercises 5.1 and 5.2 again now to see if there is any change in your beliefs about who is responsible for sexual abuse? Even a small change means you are beginning to challenge the beliefs you have held for so long. Don't worry if you have completed the exercises in this chapter and you still think the abuse was your fault. The chapter on abusers will help you to continue working on who is responsible for the abuse and on regaining your power in relation to the abuser. You may also benefit from talking it through with a friend or a support person or by contacting a telephone help-line. Come back to this chapter later and try the exercises again.

The three chapters in this section have focused on challenging your beliefs that you were to blame for the abuse and on shifting the responsibility for the abuse to the abuser where it belongs. The next section helps you to explore and process your feelings towards the people who were around at the time of the abuse – the abuser, your mother or other non-abusive care-giver, and yourself as a child.

III
Feelings About Yourself and Others

This section helps you focus on your relationship with, and feelings towards, significant figures in your childhood:

- Your abuser (Chapter 8).
- Your mother or main non-abusing carer (Chapter 9).
- Yourself as a child (Chapter 10).

8
Abusers

The exercises in this chapter are aimed at helping you to understand more about your feelings towards your abuser and to begin to feel empowered in relation to your abuser. Your abuser may have been a man or a woman, a family member, a neighbour, someone you knew because of their job (e.g. a priest, social worker, teacher), a friend of the family or a stranger. Your abuser may have been a lot older than you or of a similar age. You may have regular contact with your abuser, you may have no idea where he or she is now, or your abuser may be dead. You may have had one abuser, many different abusers or have been abused by a group of people. The abuse may be still happening. Whatever the situation was then, and whatever the circumstances are now, these exercises are for you.

Working on the exercises about abusers can bring up many different thoughts and feelings. Be prepared for strong feelings to come up and make sure you know how you will cope if this happens. Many Survivors still feel powerless in relation to their abuser and may experience feelings of fear or terror when they begin to think about him or her. You therefore need to think carefully about when and where it feels safe to do these exercises. Go back to Chapters 1 and 3 and decide who you can contact and what coping strategies you will use if you need to. Approach these exercises with special care if you have a problem with flashbacks or if you see or hear your abuser when he or she is not there. The exercises could trigger these experiences, so first make sure you have worked through the exercises in Chapter 4 on dealing with flashbacks and hallucinations and feel confident about handling your reactions. Try to keep in mind that you are an adult now and have more power than when you were a child.

If you have had more than one abuser photocopy the exercises first and repeat the exercises for each abuser. It may help to start with the abuser you feel least fearful of.

Feelings towards your abuser

The first two exercises provide different ways to help you explore your feelings towards your abuser. You may wish to work through one or both exercises.

EXERCISE 8.1   TALKING TO A CHAIR

Aim   To help you express your feelings to your abuser and to feel more empowered.

Sit on a chair and pick another chair to represent your abuser. Place this chair opposite you at whatever feels the most comfortable distance. Imagine this chair is your abuser. You are able to talk to your abuser but he or she is not able to speak back to you. Talk to your abuser and tell him or her whatever you want to. Start by telling your abuser what he or she has done to you and how it has affected your life. Be aware of how you are feeling. You may experience one type of emotion most strongly – anger, love, fear, hate, upset, pity, distaste – or many different emotions mixed together. Accept whatever feelings come up and express these feelings to your abuser.

Make a note below of any feelings that came up when you were talking to your abuser.

_____
_____
_____
_____
_____
_____
_____
_____
_____
_____
_____

Example
Wakefield Survivors' feelings towards their abusers:

hate	disappointment	pity	loathing
nothing	sorry for him	rage	terror
warmth	despise him	protective	ashamed of her
anger	compassion	revulsion	forgiving
fear	murderous	love	disgust
indifference			

Survivors' comments

I felt anger, repugnance, fear, pity, revenge and power while I was doing this exercise. I allowed myself to feel like this. It helped me get it off my chest. Don't hold anything back, you can censor it or discard it later. MAYA

Even though I am post-therapy this exercise was useful as it let me know where my feelings are at the moment. Even though I have worked through the anger stage of my recovery I realized that I still have a problem with feeling responsible for my abuser's happiness. CATHERINE

Fear was the most powerful feeling I got but the more I talked the more I realized there is no way he can hurt me anymore. I am an adult now not a child. I can show him that he does not frighten me anymore. LESLEY-LEIGH

There is no right or wrong way to feel about your abuser. Allow whatever feelings you have to surface; you may be surprised by what you discover. Survivors often have a mixture of different feelings about their abusers. They may have feelings of hatred towards the abuser and also feelings of love or a desire to protect him or her, especially if the abuser is someone close, such as a family member. Other people might try to tell you how they think you should feel towards your abuser. You might also tell yourself how you ought to feel rather than simply accepting how you do feel. It can be difficult to admit to yourself or to other people that you love someone who has done awful things to you. It can also be difficult to admit to feelings of anger or hatred towards your abuser particularly if he or she is a close family member. However, it is more helpful to understand how you are actually feeling rather than to try to force yourself to feel a certain way. Some Survivors, particularly Survivors with strong religious beliefs, feel they should forgive their abuser and try to bury their feelings of anger in order to do this. This can be an added burden and delay the process of healing. For some Survivors, feelings of forgiveness may come in time but it is not a feeling that can be rushed or forced, nor a feeling that you can simply decide to have.

EXERCISE 8.2   LETTER TO THE ABUSER
Aim   To explore and express your feelings to your abuser and to feel more empowered.

Write a letter to your abuser using the space below. Allow plenty of time to do this exercise. This letter is **not to be sent**; it isn't a letter *for* the abuser but a way of working on your own feelings. Write whatever comes into your head. You may want to describe the things the abuser did to you, and how it made you feel at the time. You may want to tell him or her how the abuse affected your life as you got older and how you feel about him or her now. You don't

129

have to begin the letter with 'Dear'. Some Survivors do not want to address their abusers in this way. Start the letter in whatever way feels most comfortable.

DO NOT SEND THIS LETTER to your abuser. Doing these exercises can sometimes make Survivors start to feel strong and powerful and it can be very tempting to want to act on these feelings. However, confronting your abuser by letter or in person can have all sorts of consequences which can be extremely difficult to handle and can leave you feeling disempowered. Remember this exercise is designed to help you work on your own feelings. It is for you alone; it isn't about trying to communicate with your abuser or getting a response from him or her.

Examples
Lesley-Leigh's letter
(Lesley-Leigh was sexually abused by her brother.)

You bastard, I wish I had a gun. I want to kill you for what you did to me. Try putting your dick in my mouth now and you will not have one left. You got a lot out of hurting someone smaller than you but now I am an adult and I can stand up for myself. You will never hurt me again. You took my childhood away from me and made me feel things a child should never feel. If I hear that you have hurt anybody else the way you hurt me I will make your life a mess just like you have made mine.

Nina's letter
(Nina was sexually abused by the matron of a children's home.)

You creep. I don't know what else to class you as. You are not an animal – they have feelings, you don't. I want to tell you how you made me feel when you did those awful things to me. I felt like a robot at times. You would never let me show any emotion. You wanted to control me, even my thoughts. You never considered how you made me feel. Can you remember how you would touch me and put things in me. You knew I didn't like it, you knew I was very frightened, but you continued just to please yourself. You would use your cigarette to burn me and know it was hurting but still you never stopped. How do you think I felt? I felt used and dirty. I didn't have a mind of my own. You would say things to make me feel bad about myself. You wanted to make me feel worthless, that I was a nobody and you succeeded. I didn't like myself. I felt I shouldn't breathe the same air as other people. You made me feel so useless, not worthy to be a human person. I would let people do what they wanted and never speak up for myself. You made me feel that and I hate and detest you for it.

I am writing this letter to you but it isn't for your benefit. This is so I can let you know what kind of a creep you are. Also to let you know that you haven't destroyed me. In fact I am a stronger person. I have survived. I will never forgive you for what you did. Not just me but the other kids as well. It makes me feel cleaner getting you out of my system. I will carry on fighting until I get you out of my system forever. Soon you will be nothing. I'll be back because I haven't finished with you yet.

Maya's letter
(Maya was abused by her mother, other family members and also by a market trader.)

To the sad, sick, market trader who abused me:

I expect you felt powerful when you forced your horrible tongue into my mouth until I couldn't breathe. I should have bitten it off. Even after all this time I am afraid of having dental treatment because it reminds me of what you did. And groping me with your disgusting mucky hands. How dare you defile me with your filth?

This letter is to give you back all the bad feelings, the guilt, shame and fear that isn't mine. I now absolve myself of these things and place them firmly back where they belong – with you. I despise you.

Maya

Graham's letter
(Graham was sexually abused by his mother.)

Mother,

For as long as I remember I have wanted to say exactly what I thought of you. Obviously I left it too long as you are now dead and I didn't get the chance to ask you 'why me?' I always knew you didn't like me from a very early age even to the point of hating me. I don't know what I did to deserve the treatment I got but I know you won't rest in peace, you don't deserve to. The hatred and anger I have for you is overwhelming. I am grateful, however, that you are not here to abuse my children and to be perfectly honest I am glad they never knew you. I often ask why I had to have you for my mother. Why didn't you have me adopted? I most likely would have had a better life and not been beaten or treated like a dog, but you couldn't even do that for me. I am now an adult but you left me scarred. Instead of beating me you should have loved me but your only priority was your next pint. I should have been able to come to you for help and advice and not a kick in the teeth. I want to forget you but the effect you had on my life has been too great. I know I put too much energy into hating you but you are not going to ruin my marriage or my children because I won't let you. I won't even visit your grave because you don't deserve my tears. I won't cry for you and I won't let you ruin the rest of my life. I want to live my life for me.

Survivors' comments

It gave me confidence to express myself without apologizing. I felt some fear while I was completing the exercise but I carried on writing and felt stronger afterwards. I felt satisfied with the results. Giving the feelings back felt good. Go for it! Tell yourself you can do it. MAYA

I found this a very powerful exercise – once I got writing the thoughts just seemed to flow. It would be easy to blank out the memories for the sake of other members of the family. But it is important for me to have a reminder of the extent of the damage caused to me and how it affected my life. I tend to try and please others. This letter helped me to put my thoughts straight and to feel that I am still managing to put myself first and to feel empowered against my abuser. I feel much more confident writing my thoughts rather than talking aloud. Seeing my thoughts written down makes them much more real than just words floating in the air. I think having written a letter it could be tempting to post it. Don't do it – you'd regret it later. CATHERINE

Say what you really feel, don't hold anything back. It's important! REBECCA

Standing up to your abuser in imagination

The exercises in the next section aim to help you overcome feelings of fear about your abuser and to feel more empowered. They also help to reinforce the knowledge that what happened to you was not right and that you were not to blame for being abused. Before you start it is important to keep in mind that all these exercises are to be done on paper or in your imagination, *not in person with your abuser.*

This section of the chapter is divided into four steps:

- What you would like to say to your abuser.
- How abusers usually react to confrontations and how *your* abuser might react.
- How to respond assertively to your abuser.
- An imaginary confrontation with your abuser.

Confronting your abuser *in imagination* can be a very powerful and liberating experience for Survivors. Confronting your abuser in person is a very different matter and can be dangerous to you, both physically and psychologically. These exercises are *not* aimed at helping you confront your abuser in person but at helping you understand more about your own thoughts and feelings about the abuse and the abuser. *Do not use the exercises below face to face with your abuser.*

1   What do you want to say?

Think about what you would like to say to your abuser if you got the opportunity to and if you felt strong and powerful enough to say anything you liked. Think about what you said in Exercise 8.1 and what you wrote in exercise 8.2. Do you want to express how you feel about the abuse or about your abuser? Do you want to tell the abuser how he or she has damaged your life?

EXERCISE 8.3   WHAT DO YOU WANT TO SAY?
Aim   To think clearly about what you would like to say to your abuser as a first step towards confronting your abuser in imagination.

Write down below anything you would like to say to your abuser as a series of brief statements.

133

What I want to say to my abuser.
e.g. You masturbated in front of me when I was a child and I am very angry with you.

I have an eating problem now because you raped me as a child.

_____

_____

_____

_____

_____

_____

_____

_____

_____

_____

_____

Catherine's example

You belted my brother I heard you. You made me live in fear.
I heard mum crying in the night and you shouting at her.
You touched me between my legs while smiling at me and telling me it was
  nice.
Because of you I became anorexic, bulimic and regularly slashed my arms.
The effects of your abuse of me lasted 20 years – think about that.
I was 3 years old and had done nothing to deserve any of this.

2   Abusers' reactions

When abusers are confronted about the abuse in person they rarely admit to what they have done. They usually **deny** that the abuse ever happened or **minimize** what really happened by pretending it wasn't sexual abuse but something innocent or loving. Some abusers **blame** the Survivor for what happened, often by suggesting the Survivor wanted the abuse or caused it to happen in some way – these may be the same things the abuser said to the Survivor as a child. Some abusers **threaten** the Survivor for speaking about the abuse and again this may be a familiar pattern from childhood. Abusers might also try to make the Survivor feel sorry for him or her by making **excuses** or talking about their own problems and try to **guilt-trip** the Survivor into remaining silent. Abusers might also try to confuse the Survivor or divert the conversation by throwing in **red herrings**, for example by challenging details of what has been said or expecting the Survivor to prove what he or she has said.

We give an example of each of these types of reactions below:

Denying	I don't know what you're talking about.
Minimizing	I was only tickling you.
Blaming	You got into bed with me.
Threatening	No one will speak to you again.
Excusing	I was under a lot of stress at the time.
Guilt-tripping	You know I'm not in good health. Why are you being so nasty to me?
Red herrings	You say I did these things in my car! Then tell me what sort of car it was.

Understanding more about the ways abusers try to deny or minimize the abuse, and blame, threaten or confuse their victims, and naming these reactions, helps you step back and see more clearly your abuser's responsibility for the abuse.

EXERCISE 8.4   MY ABUSER'S REACTIONS

Aim   To anticipate how your abuser might react if you challenged him or her as a second step towards confronting your abuser in imagination.

Think about how your own abuser might react if you said the things you wrote down in Exercise 8.3, and write these reactions below as short statements.

Abuser's reactions

e.g. You kept taking your clothes off in front of me

3 Responding assertively to your abuser

Learning how to challenge abusers' reactions by responding assertively (in the exercise, not in person) can help you feel more in control and more powerful in relation to your abuser.

Below are some examples of abusers' reactions and in the right-hand column are examples of how to respond assertively to each of these types of reactions.

Abusers' reactions	Assertive response
Denying	
I don't know what you're talking about	Yes, you do, you made me touch your penis
You are mad/a liar	No I am not mad/a liar. You masturbated on to me
I did no such thing	Yes you did. You fondled my breasts
Minimizing	
I was only tickling you	You did not only tickle me, you put your fingers in my vagina
I was only cuddling you and being affectionate	You were not being affectionate, you anally raped me
Blaming	
You got into bed with me	Yes I did but I was a child. You raped me and that is your responsibility
You had an erection. You wanted it	Yes I had an erection. That is a natural response to being masturbated but you were abusing me and you are responsible
Threatening	
No one will speak to you again	I am not to blame, you are responsible. You forced me to perform oral sex
I'll tell your partner what you did	You are responsible for the abuse. I am not to blame
Excusing	
I was under a lot of stress at the time	You may have been under a lot of stress but that does not excuse the fact that you were an adult and you masturbated in front of me

Abusers' reactions	Assertive response
Guilt-tripping	
You know I'm not in good health. Why are you being so nasty to me?	I am not being nasty, I am stating the truth. You buggered me when I was a child and you are responsible for what you did
I've had a lot of experiences in my life too but I don't make a fuss about it	You may have had bad experiences but that does not give you the right to masturbate me. I have every right to make a fuss about what you did to me
Red herrings	
You say I did these things in my car! Then tell me what sort of car it was	I am not here to talk about cars. You raped me and you are responsible

How to respond assertively

- Keep your replies short and simple.
- Deny anything that is untrue in what the abuser has said.
- State clearly what is true.
- Be specific about what the abuser actually did, e.g. 'You put your finger in my bottom', rather than, 'You sexually abused me'.
- Do not get drawn by irrelevant details – say they are irrelevant.

Remember. You are not trying to prove what happened but to make a clear statement about what you know happened and to express your feelings. Whatever the circumstances a child is never to blame for being sexually abused. You are the victim of a crime and the abuser could still be prosecuted for that crime no matter how long ago it happened.

EXERCISE 8.5   RESPONDING ASSERTIVELY TO YOUR ABUSER IN IMAGINATION

Aim   To think of assertive responses to your abuser's imaginary reactions as a way of feeling more empowered and as a third step towards confronting your abuser in imagination.

1   Below there are more examples of ways in which abusers might react if challenged about what they have done. Write an assertive response to each of these reactions in the right hand column. Keep your replies simple. Remember simply to deny what isn't true and state what is true. Look back at the examples for ideas about how to reply.

Abuser's reactions	Assertive response
You are sick in the head	
I was only loving you	
I was teaching you the facts of life	
You enjoyed it	
You didn't say 'No'	
You'd better be careful what you say or else	
I've had a hard life	
I've already had one heart attack, you are going to give me another	
We weren't living in that house when you were seven	

2   Write down your abuser's reactions (from Exercise 8.4) in the left-hand column and for each of your abuser's reactions write down an assertive response. Try to be as specific as you can in saying what the abuser did to you, e.g. 'You made me suck your penis', rather than, 'You sexually abused me'. Don't get side-tracked by irrelevant details (red herrings), for example, arguments about when certain things happened in your childhood.

Abuser's reactions	Assertive response

_____   _____
_____   _____
_____   _____
_____   _____

Examples

Abuser's reactions	Assertive response
Catherine's example	
I loved you	That is irrelevant
You probably would have had problems anyway	No. Your abuse caused me these problems
Anthony's example	
I don't know what you are talking about	Yes you do and it is no good denying it. You touched me by playing with my penis
You are a liar	There is only one liar here and it ain't me
You enjoyed it as much as I did	No I did not enjoy it at all. If I reacted to you touching my penis or other parts of my body it is because that is a normal reaction
You kept taking your clothes off in front of me	That is normal. When you are a child you take your clothes off in front of someone when you are getting ready for bed or going in the bath. I was not asking to be abused at all but you abused me
Lesley-Leigh's example	
You didn't look like a child	I was well developed but I was still a child
You deserved what you got	Nobody deserves to be abused and frightened like I was

Survivor's comment

Because it was so concise this felt like an empowering exercise. I felt I could put the abuser back where he belonged. It also helped to confirm in my mind that the abuse did happen. CATHERINE

4   Imaginary confrontation

Now you can try to put the whole thing together and try an imaginary confrontation with your abuser. *This is an exercise only and not to be done face to face with your abuser.*

Remember:

- State what is true and say what isn't true.
- Don't get drawn into arguments about irrelevant details.
- Keep repeating what you know to be true whatever the abuser's reaction. This is the 'broken record' technique – you keep saying the same thing again and again like a record where the needle is stuck.

Below we describe three ways in which you can do this. You can choose the method that suits you best or try them all.

EXERCISE 8.5   ROLE-PLAY CONFRONTATION

Aim   To role-play a confrontation with your abuser as a way of feeling more empowered in relation to him or her and of challenging negative reactions to yourself.

Chair role-play

- Get two chairs, one to represent yourself and one to represent your abuser as you did in Exercise 8.1. Place them at a comfortable distance apart.
- Sit in the chair that represents you and speak to your abuser. Say the things you would like to say if you could – the things you have written down in Exercise 8.3.
- Swop chairs and talk back to yourself as if you are your abuser using your abuser's reactions you wrote down in Exercise 8.4.
- Return to your own chair and reply to your abuser as yourself using the responses from Exercise 8.5.
- Continue swapping chairs and confronting your abuser until you feel ready to stop.

Remember you are in charge of this conversation and can stop it whenever you want to.

Role-play with a friend

Ask a trusted person if they will help you role-play a confrontation with your abuser. Talk to your friend about the work you have been doing in this chapter or ask them to read this chapter. Make sure they understand what sorts of things you want to say to your abuser, the range of ways in which the abuser might react, and how to respond assertively to these reactions.

Now role-play the confrontation with your friend. If your friend is able to make good assertive responses it may help if you start by playing the abuser and let your friend play you. Once you have done this, swop roles so your friend plays the abuser and you play yourself.

Role-playing can be a very powerful experience. Agree with your friend before you begin that you both have the right to stop the role-play at any point if you want to. At the end of the role-play remind yourselves who you really are and spend some time talking about ordinary things.

Record below your feelings and thoughts about the conversation with your abuser. You may want to record details of the conversation as a reminder to yourself.

_____
_____
_____
_____
_____
_____
_____
_____
_____
_____

EXERCISE 8.6 WRITTEN CONFRONTATION

Aim To write a confrontation with your abuser as a way of feeling more empowered in relation to him or her and of challenging negative reactions to yourself.

Use what you have written in Exercises 8.3–8.5 as the starting-point to write a confrontation between you and your abuser. Write the confrontation in the form of a play or dialogue. For example:

Me   You raped me when I was 8.
Abuser   I don't know what you are talking about.
Me   There is no use trying to deny it. You raped me when I was a
          child and you are responsible. What you did was very damaging
          to me and illegal.

_____
_____
_____

_____
_____
_____
_____
_____
_____
_____
_____
_____
_____
_____
_____

Example of Graham's role-play confrontation

I felt very sad and at the same time frightened. I began to feel my body pulsate and I was trembling. I knew my abuser was dead but I began to tell her how she and the other bastards had screwed up my life. I knew that I had the *power* to get rid of her and could shut her off at any time I wanted. I began to feel very emotional and I could feel the tears build up. I did not break down and cry and fight against it. I asked her if she thought I was so bad that she did the things she did and let others do it. She said she did nothing to me and she said I was still the lying little bastard I had always been. I could feel the anger build up and my head felt like it was going to explode rather like a balloon.

The next time I did the exercise I told her assertively that she was responsible along with the other bastards who repeatedly raped and abused me. I said: 'I am sick of living my life believing it was my fault. Do you know I fucking hate you and I am glad you are dead. I never wanted to do those things that you made me do. I only did it willingly because I could not take the beatings if I didn't. All this *is* your fault because you fucking started it. Go away and leave me and my family alone.'

At first I was really scared but then I asked myself, 'Why?' I think I saw a person so pathetic that my feelings were slowly gradually getting better and stronger. For the first time in 35 years I can see that although I was a child then, I am not a child anymore. GRAHAM

Survivors' comments

Today the world looks very different. Now I no longer immediately blame myself if things go wrong. I am able to step back and look at the situation from the perspective of 'I'm OK' and able to assess my part in the problem. REBECCA

With my brother as the abuser I found it very hard to keep doing this exercise because the fear I felt with my brother was too much for me. I was very frightened of my brother but I was also very mad because he hurt me and he had no right to do that to me. Doing the confrontation exercise about my uncle was different. I felt more in control which was nice. LESLEY-LEIGH

Standing up to other people about the abuse

It is not only abusers who react negatively when Survivors speak out. You may have tried to talk about the abuse to family members, friends or people you thought might help you but had unhelpful reactions that left you feeling confused, guilty, upset or angry. Perhaps they didn't believe you or minimized what happened. Perhaps they blamed you for the abuse or tried to make you feel sorry for the abuser and guilty for speaking out. Learning to assert yourself about the abuse with other people can also be empowering and help to contribute to breaking the hold your abuser has over you. You can use the confrontation exercises above to practise asserting yourself with others. Anthony used the written confrontation to assert himself (in imagination) with his auntie about being abused by his uncle (her brother).

Example of Anthony's written confrontation with his auntie

Me   I don't like confronting you with this but you already know that I have been to the police and made a statement about your brother abusing me.

Auntie   Yes, I know that you have been to the police because your uncle has told me that they have had him in for questioning. I have spoken to him about him abusing you and he said he never abused you at all and he thinks the world of you and there is no way he could hurt you in that way.

(Denial)

Me   Well he did and he has caused me a lot of pain and suffering over the years because when it happened I was only a child.

Auntie   So why have you waited this long if it did happen when you were a child? Why didn't you tell anyone then? **(Blaming)**

Me   Because I was so scared that no one would believe me and when it first started I was too young to know about the facts of life.

Auntie   But when you did know about the facts of life how come you let it carry on? By then you should have known that he was doing something wrong to you so you should have stopped it then. **(Blaming)**

Me   But I was so ashamed of myself for letting it carry on for so long and I wondered what the consequences would be – would you say that I was as guilty as him? Also he still had power over me because when you are in

	your teens you are still a boy and he was an adult with adult authority over me and you are told to trust your elders. Can you understand that?
Auntie	Yes, I know that you are told to trust your elders. But where is going to the police going to get you? Can't you just let it drop and forget about it? You know if proceedings go ahead he may end up in Stanley Royd [a psychiatric hospital] again. **(Guilt-tripping)**
Me	Don't forget that he has been pulled in by the police before for abusing children and he didn't end up in Stanley Royd then.
Auntie	Because they didn't press charges against him because they had no proof that he had been abusing. **(Red herring)**
Me	Well he abused me and I wouldn't lie about that and I think he must have abused others. So put yourself in my shoes knowing that he has abused and that he has caused a lot of pain and suffering and that he could still be abusing some child or teenager.

Challenging your own negative thoughts

Survivors who have had their abuse denied or minimized by their abuser or other people or have been blamed or threatened often believe what they have been told. What has been said to them is what they learn to say to themselves. You may pretend that the abuse didn't happen (**denying**) or think that it wasn't that bad (**minimizing**). You may be repeating to yourself what the abuser and others have said to you but denying and minimizing can also be a way to cope with the painful reality of your experiences. You may **blame** yourself for the abuse – thinking you caused it to happen or should have stopped it. You may also be **excusing** the abuser and be **guilt-tripping** yourself about the distress others might feel if you speak about the abuse. Survivors who have been threatened by their abuser often believe that the threat will be carried out if they talk about the abuse. They may internalize their abuser's threats and in a way may now be **threatening** themselves into remaining silent. You may, for example, be thinking that if you speak out you will die or that something terrible will befall your family or that the abuser will know and punish you. Sometimes Survivors' fears that the threats will come true result in hallucinations of their abusers.

You can use the confrontation exercises to confront your own negative thoughts and to respond assertively to them. Instead of confronting your abuser, use the exercises to confront the part of yourself that is denying, minimizing, blaming, excusing, guilt-tripping and threatening. Write down your own negative thoughts, e.g. 'I got into bed with him', on the left side of the page and an assertive response on the right. Learning to identify and challenge what you are saying to yourself can change your beliefs and help you break the internalized power of your abuser.

This chapter helps you focus on your feelings towards your abuser and to be clear about your abuser's responsibility for the abuse. The exercises build up step-by-step to a confrontation exercise with your abuser in imagination. Standing up to your abuser in imagination is a way of feeling more empowered and breaking free from the hold he or she still has over you in your mind. The exercises in this chapter can also help you to stand up to other people about the abuse, and challenge your own negative thoughts. The next two chapters help you to continue to work on issues with others (Chapter 9 Mothers) and yourself (Chapter 10 Childhood).

9
Mothers

Survivors frequently have strong negative or confusing feelings about people who were around them and didn't protect them from the abuse. These feelings are often directed towards their mothers, but may be directed to other people who did not sexually abuse them and who were supposed to be taking care of them, such as their stepmothers, adoptive or foster mothers, grandparents, fathers or aunts. In this chapter the term 'mother' is used to refer to the main care-giver who did not sexually abuse you.

Some children are sexually abused by their mothers. If this happened to you, work on your feelings towards your mother using the exercises in Chapter 8 (Abusers) and use this chapter to work on your feelings towards your other main care-giver if you had one.

The purpose of this chapter is to help you understand the difficulties you may have in your relationship with your mother and to find ways of exploring and expressing the range of your feelings towards her. We also explore why some mothers don't protect their children from abuse and how this can make children feel they weren't worth protecting. You can do these exercises even if your mother or other main care-giver is dead or if you are no longer in contact with him or her.

Relationships with mothers

Many people, whether they have been sexually abused or not, have problems in their relationships with their mothers. Childhood abuse can add specific difficulties to the child–mother relationship. The next two exercises help you to focus on your current and childhood relationship with your mother and to think about how the sexual abuse may have caused difficulties in your relationship.

EXERCISE 9.1   RELATIONSHIP WITH MY MOTHER NOW

Aim   To help you focus on the nature of your current relationship with your mother.

Read through the following list and tick off any items that apply to you.

Applies to you?

My mother or main care-giver:

- Is dead... _____
- Is alive but we are no longer in contact................ _____
- Still does not know about the abuse..................... _____
- Now knows about the abuse and
    - supports me.. _____
    - rejects the abuser.. _____
    - still lives with the abuser .... _____
    - is still in contact with the abuser.................... _____
    - does not acknowledge the abuse to me.............. _____
    - blames me for it.. _____
    - does not believe me... _____

Towards me, my mother is:

Abusive.. _____
Angry... _____
Critical/judgemental... _____
Argumentative/quarrelsome..................................... _____
Changeable... _____
Cold and distant... _____
Unsupportive.. _____
Unassertive/passive... _____
Honest and assertive .... _____
Understanding and sympathetic............................... _____
Supportive.. _____
Warm and loving.. _____

With my mother I am:

Abusive.. _____
Angry... _____
Critical/judgemental... _____
Argumentative/quarrelsome..................................... _____
Changeable... _____
Cold and distant... _____
Unsupportive.. _____

	Applies to you?
Unassertive/passive	_____
Honest and assertive	_____
Understanding and sympathetic	_____

With my mother I am:

Supportive	_____
Warm and loving	_____

Describe below in your own words your current relationship with your mother.

_____

_____

_____

_____

_____

_____

_____

_____

_____

The effects of sexual abuse on your relationship with your mother

There are many reasons why Survivors have problems in their relationships with their mothers. The sexual abuse itself can create a barrier between mother and child because abused children often feel they cannot talk about the abuse and therefore need to keep themselves at an emotional distance from their mothers. Abused children may also keep themselves at a distance from their mothers because they feel ashamed of what is happening to them and concerned about how their mothers might react if they found out about it. The relationship between a child and his or her mother may be particularly difficult if the abuser is the mother's partner. This can make the abused child feel he or she has betrayed the mother or the mother might feel jealous of the child's 'special' relationship with the abuser. Some mothers although not sexually abusive can be neglectful, uncaring or physically or emotionally abusive. This can increase the distress of children who are being sexually abused and make them feel more unloved, alone and unprotected.

EXERCISE 9.2 RELATIONSHIP WITH MY MOTHER WHEN I WAS A CHILD

Aim To describe how your mother behaved towards you when you were a child or young adult and to look at how the sexual abuse affected your relationship with her.

Below is a list of some of the ways mothers behave towards their children and a list of the specific difficulties sexual abuse can add to the relationship. Read through the lists and tick any items that applied to you. You may be able to add some others at the end.

Applies to you?

My mother was:

Absent...

Cruel and mean......................................

Physically abusive..................................

Cold and distant.....................................

Neglectful...

Showed no interest in me........................

Affectionate..

Attentive/spent time with me..................

Warm and loving.....................................

Physically affectionate............................

How the sexual abuse affected your relationship with your mother:

As a child I thought my mother knew about the abuse

I thought she was jealous of my relationship with the abuser..

I felt I was betraying my mother.............................

Keeping the abuse secret created a barrier between us .

I thought she should have protected me ....

I was scared she would find out about the abuse ....

My mother or main care-giver:

Didn't notice signs of the abuse............................

Ignored signs of the abuse....................................

Didn't listen or believe when I tried to tell...............

Found out about the abuse when I was a child or a young person and

didn't believe ....

supported the abuser ....

rejected me...

blamed me ....

didn't stop it...

Write down any other difficulties relating to the sexual abuse which may have damaged your relationship with your mother.

_____

_____

_____

_____

_____

_____

_____

_____

Having described your current relationship with your mother and identified the difficulties caused by the sexual abuse, the next section helps you explore your feelings towards her.

Feelings towards your mother

Many people, whether they have been sexually abused or not, have a complex set of feelings towards their mother or mother-figure. Survivors may feel love, hate, pity, guilt, resentment or be over-protective, angry or jealous towards their mothers, or have any combination of feelings at the same time.

> Mum, I love you, I always will. But that doesn't mean I can't feel angry with you and let down by you. CATHERINE

Survivors may feel angry towards their mothers for not protecting them or feel very protective towards their mothers and determined that they will never know about the abuse. Some of you may have spent your life trying to please your mother in order to win her approval. The complex and often conflicting feelings Survivors hold for their mothers can lead to relationship difficulties.

EXERCISE 9.3   FEELINGS TOWARDS YOUR MOTHER
Aim   To help you explore and express your feelings towards your mother.

The exercises below suggest different ways of helping you become more aware of the whole range of your feelings towards your mother. You may wish to do all three of the following exercises or one or two of them.

Letter to your mother
Write a letter to your mother expressing all the feelings you have towards her. *Do not send this letter.* The purpose of the letter is to help you become more aware of your feelings – it is not about communicating with her. It is not intended that your mother should ever see this letter, so use the opportunity to

write down how you really feel. Express all your feelings, positive or negative, and try not to judge yourself for having 'bad' or difficult feelings towards her. You may want to start by telling her why you are writing to her, how you felt about her at the time of the abuse and how you feel now.

Letter to my mother

Talking to a chair

Some people find it easier to talk rather than write. Get two chairs and sit on one of them. Imagine your mother is sitting on the other. Move the position of the chairs so that you feel comfortable. Begin talking out loud to your mother. Some people find it easier to start by talking about everyday things such as what kind of day they have had. When you feel ready tell her how you feel about her, all your feelings – positive and negative. Remember she cannot hear you, answer back or be hurt by what you say so feel free to say anything you like. It may be difficult to get going, so be patient and give yourself plenty of time.

Make some notes in the speech bubble below about what you said.

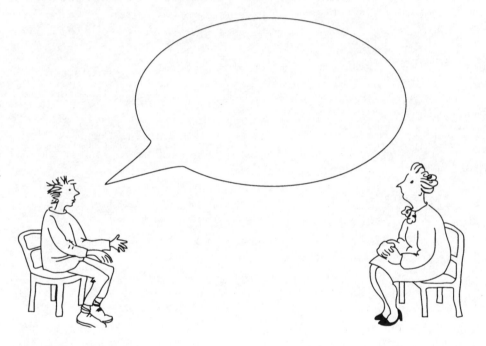

Drawing your feelings

Some people prefer to express their feelings in non-verbal ways, e.g. by drawing or painting how they feel. Think about your mother and allow yourself to express your feelings with paints, pencils, crayons, plasticine or clay, or any other art materials.

When you have done one or all of the three exercises above try sitting quietly and becoming aware of how you are feeling *now*. Stay with your feelings for a short time then find a way of expressing them. If you are sad or grieving, crying may help you release these feelings. You may feel like dancing, doing physical exercise, writing about how you feel, or contacting a friend or support person.

Example of Lesley-Leigh's letter to her mother
(Lesley-Leigh was sexually abused by her older brother and her uncle.)

Dear Mum,

I am writing this letter to you to help me deal with my own feelings towards you. For a long time I did hate you because I do believe you knew I was getting abused and you did nothing to help me. Now I feel sorry for you knowing that you have to live with the guilt for the rest of your life. It's you that has to look at my brother's face every day, not me.

You made me feel like I was not part of the family. I was the odd one out. When I was younger I hoped I was adopted because I could not believe I was hated so much. I wanted a family like my friends at school had. I would tell myself my real mother would come and get me.

When you made me have an abortion I did not know what was happening. You sent me away with a person I did not like. After a month I was allowed back home but you never asked how I felt. It was brushed under the carpet so none of the family would know anything about it. I was 12 years old for fuck's sake. I was getting blamed for something I didn't know anything about. It was when I was about 14 years old I realized that what my brother and uncle were doing to me was not right. But what could I have done, where could I have gone? You were never there as a mother for me. I just put up with it while you were in the next bedroom. Why didn't you ask me why I spent most of the night crying? You always said you were a light sleeper so how come you never heard him walk past your bedroom to come into mine? Why did you let someone hurt me? You could have stopped all the pain I went through. My childhood was taken away from me and you could have helped me.

Did you love me at all? I am glad you are out of my life but I feel that somewhere deep down inside me there is still a bit of love.

What I cannot understand is why you didn't believe me when I told you when I was 25 years old. You then turned round and said he was sleep walking. You need to make up your mind – either he did abuse me or he didn't.

The only thing I still hate you for is not showing me how to love my kids. But I now know that I will try my hardest not to treat them in the way you treated me. It is very hard but I am working on it. I am going to be a much better mother than you ever were. I am glad you are no longer part of my life.
LESLEY-LEIGH

Catherine's example of talking to a chair
Catherine was sexually abused by her father. She imagined her mother sitting on a chair and told her how she felt about her. Here are a few of the things she said.

I love you, you'll always be my mum. You knew me better than anyone. So why didn't you ask me why I was so troubled? You must have noticed. There was such a change in me when my dad was in the house. You made a big mistake. I want you to know how angry I feel. I also want to thank you for the proper love you gave me that made me feel special.

Survivor's comment

After writing the letter to my mother I talked to a chair and I felt very angry with my mother because she wasn't there to listen to what I had to say. I got mad and kicked the chair and broke it. I got rid of a lot of anger. I suggest to other Survivors trying this exercise that if you feel angry like I did then use something softer to take your anger out on! LESLEY-LEIGH

Anger towards mothers

Some of you, like Lesley-Leigh, may find that doing these exercises has brought up strong feelings of anger towards your mother. Your mother may have abandoned you, neglected you, blamed you, not believed you or supported the abuser. She may not have noticed the abuse or she may have known it was happening but done nothing to stop it. If your mother did not look after you or protect you, you have the right to be upset and angry. Your feelings are important and you may want to continue expressing your feelings outwardly by writing, talking to a chair again, or by doing something physical like hitting a cushion or taking some exercise.

You may not have felt nurtured and looked after by your mother, so before you move on to the next exercise spend some time being kind and gentle to yourself. Find some way of looking after yourself – perhaps by having a bath with your favourite bubblebath, eating a healthy meal or giving yourself a treat.

Sometimes (non-abusing) mothers are blamed by Survivors for the sexual abuse. **The mother may be responsible for not protecting the child but the abuser is always responsible for the abuse.** The next section explores why some mothers don't protect their children.

Why didn't my mother protect me from the abuse?

> Mother, I feel mostly nothing towards you. In the past I felt a mixture of anger and pity. Maybe the pity was guilt. Guilt because I hated you. I remember when you were ill how I resented having to visit you. One day you couldn't get out of bed due to your bad back and I stood and ignored you. I couldn't bring myself to touch you. I felt so nasty because I didn't help you. Maybe I resented helping you in your hour of need because you did nothing to help me. SARAH

Some mothers do not know that their children are being abused. Others do not protect their children, do not believe them when they try to tell about the abuse, or do not stop the abuse when they are aware it is happening. This can make Survivors angry with their mothers for not protecting them or very confused, sad or perplexed about *why* they didn't protect them. Some Survivors do not know how they feel about their mothers, and others cope with their feelings by being overprotective towards their mothers. If your mother knew about the abuse, or you thought she knew, and she didn't protect you then you might feel you deserved the abuse and were not worth looking after. In this section we will be exploring why mothers or other care-givers do not protect their children and emphasizing that *all* children deserve to be protected.

Do any of the following statements apply to you?

1 My mother did not know about the abuse.
2 My mother didn't respond to signs that abuse was happening.
3 My mother knew about the abuse but did not stop it.
4 My mother didn't protect me when I told her about the abuse.

It is sometimes difficult to know if your mother did know about the abuse. You may feel sure she did know when actually she was unaware of the abuse. You may be unconsciously protecting your mother by believing she didn't know about the abuse when actually she did know. You may never know for sure if she knew or not or why she didn't act to protect you, but the next exercises help you to explore these questions.

1   Mothers who don't know

It may seem that mothers *must* know when their children are being abused, but some mothers have no idea. Abuse occurs in secret and children are told to keep it secret. Abusers can be very skilful at covering up any signs of abuse and keeping children quiet. They are also good at manipulating people so they do not suspect anything; they can persuade a child's mother that they are caring people and the child is safe with them. Children often feel so ashamed of the abuse that they try to hide it from their mothers.

> I always felt so scared and frightened. I made it my life's work that nobody would ever find out what happened to me. REBECCA

You may have realized as a child that your mother did not know about the abuse, or it may come as a shock to realize now that your mother had no idea what was happening to you. As children we expect our mothers to know how we are feeling and what is happening to us. It is hard to believe that the strong feelings you were experiencing did not show on the outside. Realizing that the abuse wasn't obvious to your mother or that she may also have been manipulated by the abuser may help you in your relationship with her.

However, you may still feel hurt or angry and think 'She *should* have known'. You may feel guilty for feeling angry or resentful towards your mother because you believe you shouldn't have bad feelings about her. All children deserve to have a safe childhood where they are protected from harm, and it is natural to feel angry with your mother if she did not protect you – even if she didn't know what was happening at the time and therefore could not have helped you. Try to become aware of the whole range of your feelings towards your mother without judging yourself. You do not need to express these feelings to her but it can help you to acknowledge them to yourself. It may also help you work through your feelings if you then express them outwardly, perhaps by doing Exercise 9.3 again.

2   Mothers who don't respond to signs of abuse

> Mum, You knew me better than anyone, you knew the real me. So why didn't you ask me why I was so troubled? You must have noticed. There was such a change in me when my father was in the house. CATHERINE

Children often do show signs that they are being abused (we will look at these 'silent ways of telling' in the next chapter); a mother may see the abuser and child in suspicious circumstances or a child may have given hints about the abuse. Why is it that some mothers don't realize or acknowledge that the abuse is happening?

EXERCISE 9.4   WHY SOME MOTHERS DON'T RESPOND TO SIGNS OF ABUSE

Aim   To help you explore the reasons why your mother didn't notice or act on signs of the abuse.

Here is a list of some of the reasons why mothers may not recognize signs that abuse is going on. You may not know if these reasons applied to your mother or not. Look through the list and tick off those that might have applied to your situation. You may be able to add some more at the end.

Why some mothers don't respond to signs of abuse

Applied to you?

The abuse always happened when my mother wasn't there.. _____

She was wrapped up in her own problems at the time and didn't notice me .... _____

She was always out of the house............................. _____

She was often ill and not around to see it................ _____

She was always drunk and didn't notice anything ...... _____

The abuser was very skilled at covering it up............ _____

She was not aware of sexual abuse or its signs.......... _____

The abuser told her I was just behaving badly............ _____

She thought the changes in my behaviour were caused by something else .... _____

The abuser told her we were just playing   ..... _____

She just thought I was a moody child..................... _____

She couldn't believe her own child was being abused – 'it only happens in other families'....................... _____

She loved the abuser and couldn't imagine he or she could do it .... _____

_____   _____

_____   _____

_____   _____

_____   _____

_____   _____

Pauline's example

Some of the abuse happened in other people's houses or 'trusted' people used to take me and my brothers out to places where they abused me. At home my mother was the victim of all kinds of abuse off my father and probably didn't even know what planet she was on. I know she was powerless where my father was concerned as were a lot of other people. My mother was unable to protect me because of her own circumstances with my father and she was trying to protect all her children from his violence and emotional abuse. I don't think the thought of sexual abuse even entered her mind. She had far bigger worries at the time – fearing for her own and her children's welfare and maybe even their lives. After doing this exercise I now believe my mother could not have known about the sexual abuse. I don't blame anybody now except the abusers themselves.

Survivors' comments

It showed me that any feelings are OK to have. I felt hurt that I wasn't protected by my mother at the time but I also felt so sorry for her because she tried to be a perfect mother and she stood by me when she could. She didn't know about the sexual abuse then and I know she has gone through hell since she found out and has felt so guilty that she didn't protect me. She has spoken to me about it and apologized and shown me how much she regrets being unaware of the abuse at the time. I forgive her with all my heart. PAULINE

It helped me see my mum's side of things and that lessened the anger I feel towards her. I feel the need to let her know I'm not angry with her anymore. CATHERINE

When children do show signs of abuse they may be quite small changes in their behaviour or very noticeable changes. The reasons why mothers do not act when their children show signs of abuse include:

- They do not notice the signs.
- They see changes in their children but misinterpret them.
- They see the signs but deny to themselves that abuse is happening.

These reasons are discussed below.

Mothers who don't notice the signs

Some mothers do not notice signs that their children are in distress. They may not have seen the signs because they were ill or not around when the abuse was happening. Other mothers were involved in abusive relationships themselves, had drug or alcohol problems, or were so wrapped up in their own problems or their own lives that they failed to notice any signs of abuse in their children.

Mothers who misinterpret signs of abuse

Catherine's behaviour changed when her father began sexually abusing her. Catherine's mother did notice the changes in her when her father was in the house but thought Catherine was frightened of him because he was an intimidating man. It never occurred to Catherine's mother that Catherine was distressed because her father was sexually abusing her. Survivors' mothers may notice changes in their children's behaviour but interpret them in many different ways without considering sexual abuse as a possible cause. They could believe a child was bed-wetting or having nightmares because of problems at school. As children, both Pauline and Catherine thought their mothers must have noticed signs of the abuse and felt angry towards them. Both their mothers noticed their daughters were upset and disturbed but believed this to be due to other circumstances in their lives. Pauline and Catherine now believe their mothers did not know about the sexual abuse when they were children. This has helped them in their current relationships with their mothers.

Public awareness of child sexual abuse is very recent and your mother may have had little knowledge or awareness about sexual abuse. She may have noticed the changes in your behaviour or mood but not recognized them as signs of abuse and was therefore not in a position to protect you.

Mothers who deny signs of abuse

People often cope with an event that feels unbearable by telling themselves it is not really happening. Most mothers would find it easier to believe 'abuse only happens in other families' than believe it could be happening in their own. Some mothers may notice signs of sexual abuse but feel unable to bear the thought that their children are being abused and so deny it to themselves. Mothers who deny abuse in this way do not act to protect their children because they are not consciously aware that abuse is happening.

Some mothers were sexually abused themselves as children but have never told anyone or received any help. They may have pushed the abuse out of their minds or persuaded themselves it hadn't happened. A mother who is denying her own abuse may find it very difficult to see that her own children are being abused. If she recognizes the abuse of her children she has to accept that she was abused as well and this may be terrifying. Mothers in this situation may be denying to themselves that their children are suffering abuse, rather than deliberately ignoring it.

If your mother did not respond to the signs of abuse, for whatever reason, you may have felt you were not worth looking after. Remember that all children have a right to a safe childhood and you also deserved to be protected as a child.

3   Mothers who know and don't stop the abuse

It may be difficult to know whether your mother didn't notice the abuse or if she did know about it and did not act. However, sometimes it is clear that mothers *do* know about the abuse. They may actually see the abuse happening or have been told about it. If your mother knew about the abuse you have probably struggled to understand why she didn't stop it. The next exercise helps you think about why your mother failed to protect you.

EXERCISE 9.5 WHY SOME MOTHERS DON'T STOP THE ABUSE

Aim To explore the reasons why mothers do not stop abuse and to emphasize that you did deserve to be protected.

Read through the following list of reasons why some mothers don't stop abuse. See if you can add some more and tick off any that applied to you.

Why some mothers don't stop the abuse

Applied to you?

She was too concerned about herself to care about
anyone else... _____

She had been abused herself and didn't realize abuse
could be stopped or she thought abuse was 'normal' _____

She was afraid of the abuser............................... _____

She felt too powerless to stop the abuse.................. _____

She didn't trust the authorities and so wouldn't tell them _____

She didn't want the abuser to get into trouble........... _____

She was financially dependent on the abuser............. _____

She was emotionally dependent on the abuser........... _____

She was scared of breaking up the family................ _____

She couldn't cope with the scandal if it came out in the
open.. _____

She didn't want to rock the boat.......................... _____

The abuser didn't have sex with her when I was being
abused .... _____

The abuser was kinder to her when I was being abused _____

She was obsessed with the abuser and would let him do
anything.. _____

She blamed me for the abuse and thought I should
stop it.. _____

She blamed me for the abuse and thought I deserved it _____

_____ _____

_____ _____

_____ _____

_____ _____

_____ _____

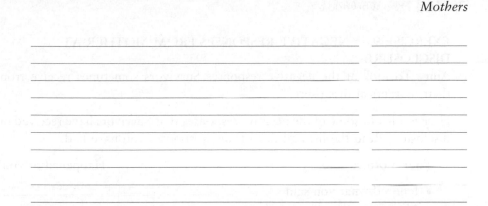

Example

> I don't think my mother knew that my uncle was abusing me because it happened at his house but I believe my mother knew I was being abused by my brother. The reasons she didn't stop it may have been:
>
> She couldn't believe her son would do something like that.
> She did not want her son to get in trouble.
> She was probably abused herself and couldn't handle it.
> She thought I'd led him on and so I deserved everything I got.
>
> LESLEY-LEIGH
>
> She couldn't see that what my stepfather was doing to me was wrong. DANNY

There are many reasons why some mothers do not stop the abuse when they know about it. All their attention and concern may have been on themselves instead of giving attention to the needs of their children. Some mothers do not feel powerful enough to stop the abuse themselves and may believe that other people are also unable to stop it. Some may turn a 'blind eye' to the abuse because they are afraid of the consequences of trying to stop it, while others may be protecting the abuser or their relationship with the abuser. Whatever the reason, it was your mother's responsibility to try to protect you.

4   Mothers who don't protect when told about the abuse

Most Survivors would not have been able to tell their mothers about the abuse. Some children and adults do tell their mothers and receive supportive and protective responses, others receive negative reactions to their disclosure. It is very damaging to both children and adults to tell and to receive a negative response and remain unprotected.

EXERCISE 9.6   NEGATIVE RESPONSES FROM MOTHER AT DISCLOSURE

Aim   To look at the negative responses Survivors sometimes receive from their mothers at disclosure.

Here is a list of some of the negative responses that Survivors have received on disclosure. Read the list and tick off any responses you have had.

Your mother:	Happened to you?

- Ignored what you said ....
- Minimized the abuse, and ....
  - said the abuser was only playing ....
  - said the abuser was tickling you......................
  - said the abuser was only being affectionate ....
- Blamed you, and...
  - slapped you ....
  - called you a slut/wicked ....
  - said you tried to steal her partner...................
  - had you taken from home so she could stay with
    the abuser (e.g. into care, hospital, to relatives) ...
  - told you to leave home...............................
- Did not believe you, and ....
  - called you a liar..
  - said you were crazy/mentally ill ....
  - said the abuser would not do anything like that....

Write down here the response you received.

_____
_____
_____
_____
_____

How did this response make you feel?

_____
_____
_____
_____
_____

Some adult Survivors believe they told their mothers about the abuse when they were children, but when they looked back at what they said they realized they had only hinted at the abuse. For example, if a child says, 'I don't like the way my stepdad plays with me,' the mother may have believed the stepfather was only playing roughly with the child. However, the child is left feeling upset that the mother did not react by protecting him or her. If you did tell, it may help you to think back to what you actually said. Pauline thought she had told her mother about the abuse by her grandfather but thinking back she realized she had not been clear:

> I didn't tell my mum properly what my grandad did to me. I was scared she might think I'd led him on. She couldn't act on what had happened because I know I wasn't direct and that I didn't tell her the whole truth.

Pauline also realized that even if she had been explicit her mother may still have been unable to protect her:

> If I had told her the whole truth she may or may not have acted on it.

Survivors often blame themselves for the abuse because they did not tell, but children are often left unprotected even after they tell.

Of course, you may have been explicit and clear but your mother still did not listen, protect you or believe you. She may have believed the abuser if he or she denied abusing. The reasons that mothers do not respond appropriately to disclosures of abuse are similar to the reasons given in the lists in Exercises 9.4 and 9.5. Look through those lists again and see if they help you understand why your mother didn't protect you when you tried to tell.

Summary: Why some mothers do not protect their children

Sometimes there are no signs that children are being abused so their mothers have no idea that abuse is happening. Where there are signs of children being upset or disturbed their mothers may genuinely believe the upset is caused by something else or not know why the child is disturbed. If your mother did not realize you were being abused then she could not protect you. However, as a child you may have felt unprotected by your mother or you may feel angry with her now; it may help you in your current relationship with your mother if you accept and work through these feelings.

Sometimes mothers take no notice of the signs, deny the abuse is happening or know about the abuse and do not stop it. Mothers who behave in these ways are responsible for not protecting their children.

If you were left unprotected you may think it was because you were not loved enough or not worth protecting. You were asked to explore why your mother didn't stop the abuse to help you understand that this was because of your mother's self-interest or situation, not because of anything you did or because you were not worth looking after. Whatever the reason, you *did* deserve to be protected.

Whether your mother knew about the abuse or not you may still be feeling sad or angry, or confused about why you were not protected. If your mother knew about the abuse or ignored the signs you may still be wondering why she did not stop the abuse. The next exercise helps you continue to explore your questions about why she didn't protect you and see if you can find some answers of your own.

EXERCISE 9.7   LETTERS TO AND FROM YOUR MOTHER

Aim   To help you understand more about why your mother did not protect you and to help you see this was because of something to do with her, not because you were not worth protecting.

Letter to your mother

Write a letter to your mother (do not send the letter) asking her why she did not protect you from the abuse. You may want to ask your mother why she didn't notice or react to any signs that the abuse was happening (e.g., any changes in your mood or behaviour, any suspicious circumstances, any hints you might have made), or why she didn't listen to or believe you if you did tell.

Your mother's situation at the time of the abuse

It may help you understand more about why your mother did not protect you from the abuse if you think about her situation at the time of your abuse. Think about the following things:

- How old was she then?
- How many children did she have?
- What other responsibilities did she have?
- Did she have a job?
- What kind of relationship did she have with her partner (if she had one)?
- What kind of relationship did she have with your abuser? (NB Her partner and your abuser may be the same person.)
- What else was happening in her life at the time?

Letter from your mother

You may now understand more about your mother's situation at the time of your abuse. Write a reply to the letter you wrote above *as if you were your mother* and write about the reasons why your mother did not notice the abuse or did not stop it. (The examples which follow this exercise may help you.)

Examples
Sarah's letters

Dear Mother,

I can come up with all kinds of reasons why you didn't protect me but, deep in my heart, I know why. You just didn't care. I was too much of a handful and you were too busy surviving your own shitty life. But I still wonder what your reasons were. Why didn't you protect me? Why didn't you love me? I know I have asked you this before and your answer was 'no one could love you, they couldn't get near you, you were a wild animal'. When you told me this didn't you ever wonder 'why'? Didn't you feel guilty?

Sarah

Dear Sarah,

I was unable to stop your abuse as I was unaware of it most of the time. I suppose I was too selfish and too busy trying to survive myself. To have acknowledged it would have caused me too much distress. I felt helpless. I know our family life was a joke but it was the only normality I knew. I didn't want to rock the boat as I had learnt a long time ago that keeping silent was the only way of keeping the family together. I pretended it was your fault and it didn't matter because you were so disturbed and damaged anyway. I am guilty of putting my need for a family before your need to be protected. I dare not acknowledge the guilt or shame because I know it will consume me and destroy my world. I would have to acknowledge that I am a failure as a mother and a human being.

Your world is so far apart from mine. What you have is what I always wanted. I want to say that I do love you and am proud to call you my daughter. I know I don't show it but that's because I know you will reject me the way I rejected you. I am sorry I did not protect you. I suffer now knowing that you do not care for me like a daughter should. You could say what goes round comes round. I have got all that I deserve.

Mother

Sarah's comments

This exercise moved me. I felt a warmth towards my mother I haven't felt before. I also felt sad writing this. I may be getting her to say what I want her to say. Maybe I'm denying or justifying my mother's actions but I realize I now understand how helpless she was. I realize that the only people to blame are the abusers.

Maya's letters

Maya was abused by her mother and felt unprotected by her stepfather. She wrote this letter to him.

To my stepfather: I know what my mother was doing to me when I was a child and so do you – no matter how much you deny it. Why on earth didn't you help me? You turned a blind eye to my abuse as you were afraid of my mother's violence and because she told you to keep out of it as I wasn't your child. How could you have colluded with her and made me feel I was bad and worthless when I loved you so much? How could you?

Dear Maya,
I know you hold me responsible for not stopping the abuse by your mother and I don't blame you. Please forgive me – none of it was your fault.

I was afraid of your mum's rages and violent outbursts, I just didn't know what to do. I thought if I stayed quiet and calm it would pacify her and sometimes it did. Your mum would cry bitterly afterwards and vow she would never hurt you again. She was very damaged by her own childhood and took it out on you.

I have many regrets about it now and wish I had done more to help you. I am truly sorry.
Love
Dad xxxxxxx

After doing these exercises some of you, like Sarah, may have more understanding of why your mothers did not notice or stop the abuse. Others may find it difficult to put themselves in their mothers' position or, like Lesley-Leigh, may not be able to think of any answers:

I have written to my mother but I cannot write back to myself from her. I feel unable to answer my questions about why she didn't protect me. I do not know the answers. No matter how I try I cannot answer them.

Lesley-Leigh's mother arranged for her to have an abortion when she was only 12 years old. Lesley-Leigh knew her mother must have known she was being raped and finds it very difficult to understand how her mother could have left her so unprotected. Some of you may never know why your mother did not stop the abuse.

It is very sad that many children are abused by a trusted adult and are not protected by their mother or main care-giver. If this has happened to you, you may be feeling sad, betrayed, confused, angry or have other strong feelings and it may help you to find your own way of expressing these feelings. **It is important to understand that you were very unfortunate to be in that situation but that it was not your fault and you did deserve to be protected. If your mother knew about the abuse and failed to protect you, for whatever reason, she is responsible for her neglect. Every child has a right to be protected from abuse.**

Changing your relationship with your mother

In this chapter we have focused on exploring your feelings towards your mother and you may now want to make changes in your relationship with her. You may understand more about her circumstances at the time of the abuse and be able to let go of resentment or negative feelings and allow yourself to have a closer or easier relationship. You may decide you want to talk to your mother about the abuse or about how you feel. This could be helpful but it could also be difficult because your mother may not believe you or respond as you expect or want her to. If you want to talk to your mother about the abuse it is important that you prepare yourself for all the possible outcomes by talking it through with someone first or role-playing what might happen.

Some mothers persist in blaming or disbelieving their children or in treating them badly. Your mother may have treated you badly over the years, and over time you may have learnt to put up with it. No one deserves to be treated badly and you do not have to accept being used or abused. Everyone has the right to decide how much contact they want with another person, including their mothers, and to choose to break off contact with someone who is abusing or upsetting them. Reducing or breaking off contact with your mother can be a painful choice and needs to be thought about carefully. However, this is a positive choice for some Survivors.

> After writing to my mother and talking to the chair I cried and felt relieved. I also felt helpless knowing she could never accept what I say. I have begun to come to terms with this and realized a happy ending is not possible. I still have occasional contact with them but I now have a separate life from my family and my mother. SARAH

It can be difficult to make changes in the important and longstanding relationship between yourself and your mother. Reading the chapter on 'Mothers' in *Breaking Free* may help you think about what you want to change in your relationship with your mother and how to approach making the changes. Receiving counselling can also help you resolve your feelings towards your mother and work on your relationship with her.

In this chapter you have explored your relationship with your mother or care-giver and perhaps become aware of how vulnerable and unprotected you were as a child. The next chapter helps you think again about your situation as a child and encourages you to look back with sympathy on the child you were.

10
Childhood

> When I was a child I used to take drugs, drink alcohol, cut myself and run away from home. The adults around me thought I was a bad child and I was behaving badly for attention. *Yes I was*, but no one asked me if I had a problem so I'd just do it even more to get more attention. Why didn't they just ask me? I needed support, care and comfort and I didn't receive any so I took drugs instead. It was love that I wanted. LESLEY-LEIGH

Children who are being abused need to find ways of dealing with their feelings and coping with what is happening to them. They often express their distress through changes in their mood or behaviour. Unfortunately adults may only see these children as behaving badly or being disruptive and may punish or blame them. The children may then come to believe that they are bad or that there is something wrong with them. Survivors can grow up thinking they were bad children as well as blaming themselves for the abuse and feeling ashamed of the sexual experiences their abusers subjected them to. As adults they often end up having negative feelings towards themselves as children, as well as thinking badly of themselves as adults.

In Chapter 2 you saw how your problems as an adult were related to your past experiences. This chapter aims to help you look back on your childhood and understand that many of your feelings and behaviours as a child were a response to the abuse. It also helps you begin to communicate with and take care of the child you were.

Many Survivors find it difficult and painful to look back on their childhoods and are afraid of being overwhelmed by feelings such as despair, loneliness, anger and shame. The exercises in this chapter help you think about yourself as a child with your current adult knowledge and understanding. It is important that you follow the suggestions in Chapter 1 and keep yourself at a safe emotional distance from your childhood experiences as you work through these exercises.

Silent ways of telling

As we discussed in Chapter 5, the majority of children do not tell anyone when they are being abused because they are manipulated by the abuser and have many other pressures on them to keep quiet. Even though they usually do not *say* anything, the behaviour of abused children often changes in some way. Children, like adults, have to find ways of coping with bad experiences and they may express their pain or confusion by, for example, wetting the bed, having nightmares, becoming moody, being disruptive at school or by eating a lot.

> As a child I was naughty and anxious and exhibited strange behaviour in the hope that people would guess I was being abused just so I didn't have to tell them and be punished for telling. EILEEN

These mood and behaviour changes can be seen as the child's silent cries for help and in *Breaking Free* we refer to them as 'silent ways of telling'. Children usually find some way of expressing their distress or crying out for help even though they cannot ask for help directly. The following exercises aim to help you become aware of the kinds of problems you had as a child and to see that you shared these problems with other children who were sexually abused.

EXERCISE 10.1   SILENT WAYS OF TELLING

Aim   To look at the ways children show they are upset or disturbed and help you see that your moods and behaviours were ways of expressing your distress.

Below is a list of mood and behaviour changes commonly displayed by abused children. If a child shows any of these problems it does not mean they have been sexually abused. The behaviours indicate that a child might be upset or disturbed by something, it may be sexual abuse or it may be any other childhood experience.

- Read through the list and see if you can add any other ways that children might express their distress or cope with abuse.
- Look back on yourself as a child. Tick off on the list any of the behaviours that applied to you. Add any of your own behaviours and feelings that are not already there.

Silent ways of telling: childhood signs of distress

The following signs suggest a child is being sexually abused:

	Applied to you?		
	Yes	A little	No
Displaying too much sexual knowledge for their age			
Inappropriate sexual behaviour, e.g. tongue kissing			
Writing stories about sex or abuse			
Drawing pictures about sex or abuse			
Sexually transmitted diseases			

The following signs do not necessarily mean a child is being sexually abused. They do indicate that something may be upsetting or disturbing the child:

	Applied to you?		
	Yes	A little	No
Eating problems			
Refusing to eat			
Overeating			
Compulsive eating			
Binge-eating			
Bingeing and vomiting (bulimia nervosa)			
Abusing laxatives			
Anorexia nervosa			
Excreting problems			
Wetting			
Bed-wetting			
Retaining urine			
Soiling			
Constipation			
Diarrhoea			
Retaining faeces			
Smearing faeces			
Changes in behaviour or mood			
Withdrawing from people			
Not communicating			
Fearful of being alone with particular people			
Not making close friends			
Trying to be perfect			

	Applied to you?		
	Yes	A little	No
Depression	_____	_____	_____
Anxiety	_____	_____	_____
Phobias	_____	_____	_____
Nightmares	_____	_____	_____
Difficulty sleeping	_____	_____	_____
Constantly tired	_____	_____	_____
Suicide attempts	_____	_____	_____
Obsessional behaviour or thoughts	_____	_____	_____
Tantrums	_____	_____	_____
Clinging to adults	_____	_____	_____
Acting younger than their age	_____	_____	_____
Running away	_____	_____	_____
Disruptive behaviour at home	_____	_____	_____
Disruptive behaviour at school	_____	_____	_____
Truancy	_____	_____	_____
Underachievement at school	_____	_____	_____
Overachievement at school	_____	_____	_____
Bullying	_____	_____	_____
Fighting	_____	_____	_____
Aggressive or violent behaviour	_____	_____	_____
Stealing	_____	_____	_____
Frequent illnesses, e.g. stomach ache, rashes, sore genitals	_____	_____	_____
Frequent 'accidents'	_____	_____	_____
Self-mutilation or self-abuse, e.g. slashing, scratching	_____	_____	_____
Alcohol, drug abuse	_____	_____	_____
_____	_____	_____	_____
_____	_____	_____	_____
_____	_____	_____	_____
_____	_____	_____	_____
_____	_____	_____	_____
_____	_____	_____	_____
_____	_____	_____	_____
_____	_____	_____	_____

Examples

Annabelle
Wanting to be thin.
Having sore throats and chest pains.
Disliking surprises.
Feeling protective of my mother.
Talking about my abuse in story form.
Avoiding sex education classes.
Being solemn.
Scared of the 'bye-bye man' who came in the night.
Always being alert/on guard.

Graham
Always apologizing.
Banging my head.
Crying and depressed.
Slashing my wrists and overdosing.
Shutting myself away.
Withdrawing from life.
No appetite.

Karen
I really wanted to be liked so I tried to be perfect. I wanted to please everyone. When I was seven I did all the housework and all the shopping. I tried to stay away from home and camped out at my friends' houses.

Lesley-Leigh
I felt I was alone. It was a way of life to let people touch you whenever they wanted to. I let boys and men have sex with me even when I didn't want to.

Danny
I used to wet my bed and I began making my bed to hide the fact because I'd get such a telling off. My mother accused me of doing it deliberately saying I was too lazy to get up in the night to go to the loo. As though I'd lay there wetting myself and lying in a pool of urine all night on purpose.
At junior school I would soil in the washbasins, on toilet seats and on the floor of the toilets.
I was stealing in and out of the home.
Extreme cases of vandalism in and out of the home.
General bad behaviour such as making false 999 calls.
Suffering intense headaches/migraines twice weekly.

Survivors' comments

> Seeing the list of 'Silent ways of telling' seemed to make my problems more acceptable because other children acted in similar ways as I did. KAREN
>
> I was reluctant to start writing. I was feeling tense and panicky at the thought of remembering what I was like as a child. I had to make myself feel safe first by waiting until I was alone in the house and climbing into my sleeping bag with my favourite cushion. I became aware of the long list of problems I had as a child and how I was crying out for help but no one heard me. I let myself feel upset and angry and managed not to space-out (my usual way of coping). It helped me understand that my behaviour as a child was an indication of my distress and not because I was bad. I feel sad that there wasn't anyone there to help me at the time. MAYA
>
> I'd not realized the extent of the problem. Doing this exercise linked together what I had regarded as separate things and a pattern formed which shows I was screaming out for help. I thought I was just a naughty boy with all this delinquent behaviour. It gave me some understanding and sympathy for my actions for which I had been labelled as bad and naughty. I felt angry at adults even ones I'd previously viewed as alright. Adults are crap, they have no idea of a child's psychology. They all bollock kids without finding out what lies behind the behaviour. No one listens to children, they're treated as second-class citizens. For teenagers it's even worse. Adults suck! DANNY
>
> I realized how many ways I'd tried to tell but I wasn't noticed. I felt upset and cried. PAULINE

Why do children behave in these ways?

Unfortunately, when children behave in the ways listed above they are often seen by the adults around them as naughty, bad, stubborn or ungrateful children. They may even be seen as 'mad'. Survivors have said that as children they were told they were: mad, bad, silly, stupid, daft, unreasonable, a spoilt little brat, evil, possessed by the devil, disruptive. Children who grow up being told these things soon begin to believe it themselves and think that their 'silent ways of telling' prove how bad they really are. They may even believe they were abused because they were bad. In fact their behaviours were ways of expressing how bad they were feeling or were ways of coping with what was happening in their lives.

EXERCISE 10.2   HOW I WAS AS A CHILD
Aim   To increase your awareness of why you felt and behaved as you did when you were a child.

- Look back on your childhood and try to see that you were *not* a bad child but a child in distress, a child who was trying to survive abuse and was crying out for help.
- Look back on your childhood and choose a time which was difficult for you. What did you think about yourself? How did you feel? How was the way you behaved affected by the abuse? Think about why you were acting in these ways and fill in the bubbles below. The examples on the following pages may help you. If you prefer write an account of how you were affected and why.

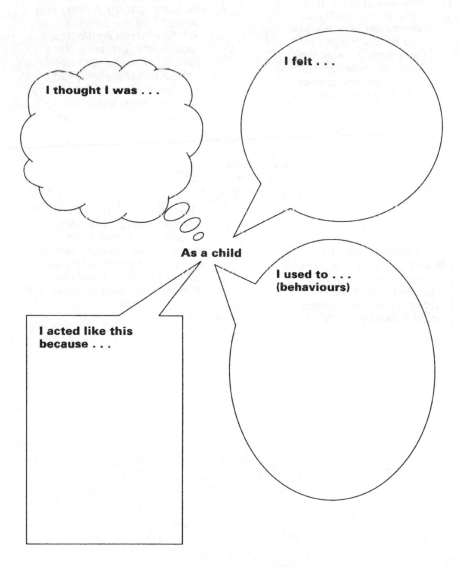

Examples

Danny

Danny was physically and emotionally abused as a child. He was taken into care because of his behaviour problems when he was 13 years old.

I thought I was . . . *an obstacle getting in the way of everything my parents did. A scapegoat for all the things that went wrong. I was their jinx, the real bane of their lives, the anchor curtailing their freedom.*

I felt . . . *fear, very big fear. Terrified of my stepfather. Often thought my mother was going to kill me (literally that is). Fearful the whole time I was in the company of my parents or in the confines of the flat. Lonely, unloved, ignored, worthless, hopeless.*

As a child

I acted like this because . . . *it was a way of expressing my inner turmoil. It was the only bit of power and control that I could get hold of.*

I used to . . . *steal from shops, friends, teachers, parents. I used to lie compulsively, make false 999 calls, throw stones at trains, motorway bridges and tower blocks, and I would smash windows.*

Maya

Maya was sexually, physically and emotionally abused by her mother. Her stepfather and the other adults around her 'turned a blind eye'.

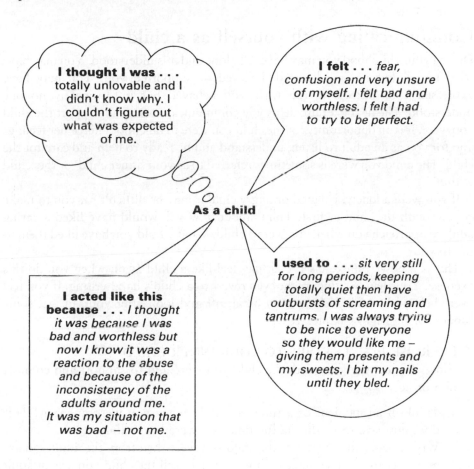

I thought I was . . . totally unlovable and I didn't know why. I couldn't figure out what was expected of me.

I felt . . . *fear, confusion and very unsure of myself. I felt bad and worthless. I felt I had to try to be perfect.*

As a child

I acted like this because . . . *I thought it was because I was bad and worthless but now I know it was a reaction to the abuse and because of the inconsistency of the adults around me. It was my situation that was bad – not me.*

I used to . . . *sit very still for long periods, keeping totally quiet then have outbursts of screaming and tantrums. I was always trying to be nice to everyone so they would like me – giving them presents and my sweets. I bit my nails until they bled.*

Survivors' comments

It helped me highlight the links between different aspects of my life. I hadn't realized how I had felt as a child or how it had had such an effect on me as an adult. DANNY

Focusing on how I felt was helpful. I don't think I have ever been asked how I felt as a child before. REBECCA

I was only three years old when I was sexually abused so I found it difficult to do this exercise. I had only feelings with no vocabulary to go with them. It did make me realize I wasn't a moody child but that I had behavioural problems due to my traumatic situation. I felt sympathy for the little girl like she was a relative I loved very much but she wasn't actually me. CATHERINE

Communicating with yourself as a child

During your childhood you may have felt alone and misunderstood. You may have tried to tell but no one listened, believed or supported you. You may have expressed your distress in the ways you behaved but unfortunately no one understood. The next exercise helps you communicate with and support the child you were. It is an opportunity for the child you were to talk about his or her feelings and for you as an adult to listen, understand and be ready to help and care for the child. The child you were is sometimes referred to as your 'inner child' or the 'child within'.

If you were a lonely, isolated or angry child it may be difficult for you to make contact with the child at first. Think about how you would have liked a caring adult to approach you when you were a child. What would you have liked them to say to you?

This is a powerful exercise. You may feel like a child again when you do this exercise. Your handwriting might even revert to a child's handwriting. If you feel overwhelmed by your feelings then break off and look after yourself, get some support or return to Chapter 1.

EXERCISE 10.3   LETTERS TO YOUR INNER CHILD
Aim   To communicate with the child you were and to support and comfort him or her.

1   Think of an incident or a time as a child when you were unhappy. This does not have to be during the time you were being abused.
    Write a letter to yourself as the child you were then from the adult you are now. Try to make contact with him or her. Tell the child you are an adult who *will* listen and believe and will try to understand what is happening. Write your letter in simple language, the sort of language a child could understand. If you had a nickname as a child you may want to use it in your letter.

Dear _____

2 Write a reply to yourself as you are now from this child. Try to remember how you felt as a child and what you would have liked from an adult. You may want to write about how you were feeling, what was happening to you, the things you didn't understand.

Dear _____

3 Continue writing letters to and from yourself as a child so the adult part of yourself is able to support and accept the child you were and the child feels comforted.

   As an adult you could try to explain to the child how he or she was not to blame for the abuse and did not deserve to be abused. The adult may be able to help the child understand his or her moods, feelings and behaviours. As you continue writing letters you may be able to get closer to the child who felt unloved and alone and offer the child love and support. You can help the child realize he or she is no longer alone. Comforting the child could take some time, so keep returning to this letter-writing exercise over the following months.

Examples

Maya's letters
Dear Little Maya,
I am so sorry for all the bad things that happened. None of them were your fault and you didn't deserve to be treated like that. I am sorry that I didn't like you before and thought you were a nuisance. That was wrong of me and I will try to make up for it now. When I look at your photograph I see a beautiful tiny child with lovely brown eyes and dimpled cheeks. I just want to pick you up and hold you, take care of you, have fun with you. We will do all of these things together. We will walk hand in hand and I will show you how lovable you are and always were.
You are not alone now.
I love you,
   Big Maya

Dear Big Maya,
Thank you very much for your letter. It means everything to me to know you care about me. I felt ugly and unwanted before. It is so lovely to be told I am beautiful and that you want to be with me. I cannot believe it yet, though, so you will have to go slowly as I am not used to trusting people.
   Little Maya

Sarah's letters
Sarah was neglected by her parents and was sexually abused by her brother and by other people outside the family. As a child she was isolated and moody. Sarah had to write several letters to her child self before the child was able to respond to her. These are extracts from some of the later letters.

Dear child,

You'll find this hard to believe but I love you and care about you. It isn't because you are no good that the people around you show no interest in you. You deserve better – they should show you kindness, understanding and warmth. To help you feel better I would like you to tell me some of the things that happened to you. I want to listen to you. I want to help you see it wasn't your fault.

Dear adult,

There are so many incidents. One time I remember was when my oldest brother would come and sit on my bed. I can remember him rubbing his tail (penis) on my privates and I felt nice. Afterwards I felt so bad I wanted to run away. I couldn't bear to see him or anyone else because of the guilt, shame and fear that someone would find out what I'd done. But I used to egg him on. I wanted him to think I wanted it even though I knew I would feel bad afterwards. It was the only time he, or anyone else, was ever nice to me. It made me feel important. I liked the attention so I was as bad as he was.

Dear child,

It was very brave of you to tell me this. Don't feel bad because you let your older brother do sexual things with you or that you received some brief pleasure. He was older and should have known better. It was your way of surviving. If you had been loved and cuddled by your family then this would probably not have happened.

Write to me again and tell me how you are feeling.

Dear adult,

I feel so miserable I don't want to get out of bed. My brothers just tease me and won't let me play. I feel so alone. I'm so angry. My mum ignores me and my dad hits me all the time.

Dear child,

It's OK to be angry – it doesn't mean you don't care about your family. Your brothers were probably being mean to you because they felt bad about what they were doing to you and didn't want to be reminded of it. Your parents are also responsible for emotionally and physically abusing you – don't be ashamed. No one will abuse you now because I will look after you. Hiding in bed won't take your feelings away but talking will help you cope with them. You can keep on writing letters to me and I will try to help you.

Survivors' comments

> I looked at a photo of myself as a child before I began, to help me 'tune in' to the exercise. I felt like a child as I wrote my letter from my inner child. As an adult again I felt compassion for the first time for the child instead of the hatred I'd always felt before. I cried and then became angry that I'd felt so bad about myself for years because of what someone else had done to me. I also felt guilt and shame for having had such strong negative feelings towards my child self. MAYA

> I felt sadness, helplessness, affection, warmth and rejection. It was too painful to think about for too long. Myself as a child is like a ghost. Writing the letters to my inner child helped me to get that bit more in touch with my childhood self. It will need several attempts before progress can be made. DANNY

> When I was writing to the inner child I felt like I was her mother and the child was someone else. I found it very hard to write to the inner child. I remembered how alone I felt as a child. It brought back a lot of feelings that I had put to the back of my mind. I coped by going for a walk then came back to it. I found I needed support from a friend. LESLEY-LEIGH

When you have finished your letters take care of yourself. First make sure you are fully back in the present. Use the grounding exercises in Chapter 4, or try Exercise 4.5 (reality orientation) if you still feel as if you are a child. You are working through this book because you had a distressing childhood so it is natural to feel upset when looking back at how you felt then.

Caring for yourself as a child

We hope you now have more understanding of yourself as a child and can see how your childhood problems related to the pain and confusion you were experiencing. You may now be able to begin to give yourself some of the care and understanding you needed as a child.

EXERCISE 10.4   CARING FOR THE CHILD YOU WERE
Aim   To help you understand and care more for the child you were.

- Find a photograph of yourself as a child. Look at the photograph and remember how you were feeling then. Think about what you would have liked from the adults around you. Keep this photograph with you, look on the child with sympathy and learn to accept the child. (If you do not have a photograph you could use a childhood toy or possession to help you remember how you felt then.)

- Think of yourself as a child and sit for a moment with your feelings. Now try to see yourself as a child. Some people find it helps them if they pick up a cushion or a soft toy and cuddle it. Imagine the cushion or toy is you as a child and see if you can give yourself some of the physical and emotional affection you needed as a child.
- Make some notes here on anything that comes up for you.

Example

When I thought of myself as a child I remember playing with my dolls, brushing their long lovely hair. I would dress up in my mother's clothes and put makeup on. What I really wanted was to have a cuddle before I went to bed. I wanted my mother to read me a story so I could fall asleep in her arms and I wanted to play my music on my own tape deck. I just wanted to be loved. Now I can begin to give the child the love she needed. LESLEY-LEIGH

Survivor's comment

I didn't have a photograph or very much left from my early childhood so I imagined myself as a small child and I held an old teddy. I realized I used to give my teddy the cuddles and talks I craved as a child. CATHERINE

It can be helpful to do this exercise regularly to allow yourself to learn to care for the child you were and for you to give the child some of the love he or she needed.

You may have felt alone and not worth looking after as a child but that is not the case now. Like many other Survivors you have taken the brave step of beginning to work on your problems and take care of yourself.

Now you have begun the process of relating better to yourself as a child it may be helpful to think about any difficulties you have now in relating to other children.

Difficulties relating to children

When someone was abused as a child or had a difficult childhood they sometimes experience difficulties in relating to children. The next exercise explores the range of difficulties Survivors commonly experience with their own or other children.

EXERCISE 10.5   RELATING TO CHILDREN
Aim   To look at the kinds of difficulties Survivors experience with children.

Below is a list of difficulties Survivors experience with children. Look through this list and tick off any that apply to you. You may be able to add some others to the list.

Difficulties with children	Applies to you?		
	Yes	No	Sometimes
Excessive fears for children's safety			
Over-protecting children			
Inappropriately protecting children			
Rejecting children			
Anger and hostility towards children			
Not being able to show love and affection towards children			
Not being able to touch children			
Controlling children			
Having difficulties with children of a certain age			
Not being able to bath children			
Having urges to abuse children			
Physically abusing children			
Emotionally abusing children			
Sexually abusing children			
Verbally abusing children			
Over-indulging children			
Being jealous of children			

Difficulties with children

	Applies to you?		
	Yes	No	Sometimes
Not being able to assert your own needs with children			
Not being able to say 'No' to children			
Feeling helpless and out of control with children			
Not feeling love for your own children			
Excessively washing children			
Unable to cope with a child feeling upset/hurt/angry			
Confusing your own feelings with the child's			

If you have physically, sexually or emotionally abused children, or have urges to do so, it is important that you seek professional help for yourself and the children you have harmed as soon as possible. The services listed in the Sources of Help section will be able to advise you.

Examples

Annabelle found she experienced several of the above difficulties and added the following:

I didn't want to have children at all and was afraid of becoming pregnant. Despite this I was reluctant to use contraception because I didn't want to acknowledge I was sexually active.

I strongly preferred having a girl to having a boy.

Maya added:

Not having empathy with children.

Not being in tune with children's needs.

Behaving erratically and inconsistently with children.

Jenny added:

Being angry with them for being vulnerable or needy.

Being unable to meet a child's needs/demands.

Survivor's comment

> I feel embarrassed that I have such negative feelings for children in general. I coped by accepting that this is how I feel although this is difficult to accept. I recognized that my feelings towards children are because of my own unmet needs. JENNY

Why do Survivors have difficulties with children?

Survivors' neediness

We have seen in this chapter how abused children often have no adult who understands how they are feeling, or no one to look after them and care about how they feel. As adults, Survivors may still be very needy themselves and this can make it difficult for them to meet the needs and demands of their own children. Survivors may also try to compensate for their own neediness by giving their children everything they didn't have themselves, even if this is not what their children need or want. Some Survivors feel jealous or resentful of children because the children are receiving love or other things they themselves were deprived of:

> I was jealous of my children having birthday parties and enjoying Christmas because I never enjoyed family activities. ANNABELLE

You have now begun to give the child you were some understanding and care. This may help you relate to other children in terms of what they need rather than what you needed as a child.

Being reminded of the abuse

Survivors often cope with their childhood abuse by burying their painful memories and feelings. Being with children can remind Survivors of their own childhood and bring back the distressing feelings and memories they have pushed away. Working through this book may help you come to terms with your past so that being with children no longer triggers bad memories.

Lack of a good parenting model

People usually learn the basic ideas of parenting from observing their own parents' behaviour. Survivors who have been abused by their parents or other care-givers may have difficulty in parenting because they have never learnt the basic skills that others take for granted. You may find it helpful to share your anxieties or concerns with other parents, read a book on childcare, attend a parenting-skills class or talk to a health visitor. Don't be afraid to ask for help or share your concerns with others.

In *Breaking Free* we discuss in more detail the difficulties Survivors experience in relating to children, and how to overcome them.

Looking back on your childhood difficulties and how you felt as a child can be painful but beginning to understand and take care of yourself as a child can help you feel better about yourself now, and may also help you in your relationships with other children. It may also help you put the past behind you and allow you to live your life in the present.

The next chapter helps you see how much progress you have made so far and helps you start to plan and look forward to your future.

IV
Looking to the Future

This section helps you assess your progress so far and helps you plan for a more positive future.

11
The Past, Present and Future

> Doing these exercises has helped me see I have come a long way from when I first started working on the abuse. I have still got things in my life that I need to deal with but I intend to face them. I have learnt that to overcome these problems we need to be honest with ourselves and those around us. LESLEY-LEIGH

This is the last chapter – congratulations on making it this far! It may have been difficult for you at times and you will probably have experienced some very powerful emotions. This chapter looks at how you have progressed in breaking free from your past and helps you assess your present position and make plans for your future. The chapter is divided into four sections:

- How have I changed?
- Maintaining progress and coping with relapses.
- What I still want to do.
- The next step.

How have I changed?

After working through this book some Survivors will have changed a great deal whereas others may feel they have not changed much at all. Each person makes changes at the right time and at the right pace for him or her. You may have changed the way you think about your past and about yourself, but your feelings may take longer to change. Sometimes it can be hard for you to see the progress you have made:

> Ask others to tell you how far you have come if you cannot remember. Other people can see changes in us that we don't – write down what they say and keep it. REBECCA

The exercises in this section help you become aware of any changes you have made in your beliefs, feelings, symptoms, coping strategies and relationships. Moving on and making progress does not mean overcoming all your problems; it does mean taking a few steps towards your future. It may mean you feel a little less guilty about the abuse, or that you binge and vomit less frequently. You may still feel depressed but not all the time now or not quite so deeply. Everybody has times when they feel low or revert to old ways of thinking or behaving. It is common to have bad days, and on bad days everything seems to look worse than usual. To get a more realistic picture of how you have moved on avoid working through this chapter on a bad day.

> When I first tried these exercises I was having a bad day and I couldn't remember how I had changed. Don't do them when you are having an 'off' day. Do the exercises in this chapter from a position of strength. Allow it to be the truth. REBECCA

EXERCISE 11.1 HOW HAVE I CHANGED? BELIEFS ABOUT ABUSE

Aim To help you see whether you have made any changes in your beliefs about who is responsible for sexual abuse.

Look through the following list of beliefs and for each one ask yourself: 'How much do I believe this right now?' Choose the number which corresponds with how much you believe each one. For example:

- If you don't believe it at all circle 0.
- If you are unsure circle 5.
- If you totally believe it circle 10.

	Don't believe at all	?	Totally believe
I could not stop the abuse because the abuser had power over me	0 1 2 3 4 5 6 7 8 9 10		
There are good reasons why I couldn't tell anyone	0 1 2 3 4 5 6 7 8 9 10		
I was abused because an abuser had access to me not because of anything I had done	0 1 2 3 4 5 6 7 8 9 10		
Abusers are always responsible for abusing children	0 1 2 3 4 5 6 7 8 9 10		
I know my abuser was responsible for abusing me	0 1 2 3 4 5 6 7 8 9 10		
The abuse was definitely not my fault	0 1 2 3 4 5 6 7 8 9 10		

	Don't believe at all	?	Totally believe
If you had more than one abuser:			
I had more than one abuser because several abusers had access to me	0 1 2 3 4 5 6 7 8 9 10		
I had more than one abuser because I was in a vulnerable and unprotected situation	0 1 2 3 4 5 6 7 8 9 10		

When you have completed this exercise you may want to compare your answers with those you gave in Exercise 5.2 to see if you made any changes in your beliefs about abuse as you worked through this book. Every small step towards feeling less guilty is an important step forward.

Survivor's comment

I believe I have gained my power back from my abusers. The knowledge I have now makes me feel so strong. The more you recognize where the blame lies the better you feel and the stronger you get. PAULINE

EXERCISE 11.2   HOW HAVE I CHANGED? FEELINGS ABOUT MYSELF
Aim   To rate how you feel about yourself now.

Look through the following list of statements and circle the number which corresponds to how much you agree with each one. For example:

- If you totally agree with it then circle 0.
- If you neither agree nor disagree then circle 5.
- If you totally disagree then circle 10.

Feelings about myself	Agree	?	Disagree
I hate myself	0 1 2 3 4 5 6 7 8 9 10		
I don't like myself	0 1 2 3 4 5 6 7 8 9 10		
I feel worthless	0 1 2 3 4 5 6 7 8 9 10		
I don't accept myself	0 1 2 3 4 5 6 7 8 9 10		
I am bad	0 1 2 3 4 5 6 7 8 9 10		
I do not like the child I was	0 1 2 3 4 5 6 7 8 9 10		
I do not feel positive about the future	0 1 2 3 4 5 6 7 8 9 10		
I feel helpless	0 1 2 3 4 5 6 7 8 9 10		

EXERCISE 11.3   HOW HAVE I CHANGED? MY RELATIONSHIP WITH MY FEELINGS

Aim   To look at how you relate to your feelings now.

Look through the following list of statements and circle the number that corresponds to how much you agree with each one. For example:

- If you totally agree with it then circle 0.
- If you neither agree nor disagree then circle 5.
- If you totally disagree then circle 10.

My Feelings	Agree					?					Disagree
I am overwhelmed by my feelings	0	1	2	3	4	5	6	7	8	9	10
I am not in touch with my feelings	0	1	2	3	4	5	6	7	8	9	10
I am frightened of my own feelings	0	1	2	3	4	5	6	7	8	9	10
I am cut off from my feelings	0	1	2	3	4	5	6	7	8	9	10
I am ill at ease with my feelings ..	0	1	2	3	4	5	6	7	8	9	10

You may want to compare your ratings now with how you answered the same exercises (2.2 and 2.3) earlier in the book to see if you feel a little better about yourself now or feel more comfortable with your own feelings.

EXERCISE 11.4   HOW HAVE I CHANGED? SYMPTOMS AND COPING STRATEGIES

Aim   To help you become aware of any reductions in your symptoms or any positive changes in your use of coping strategies.

Think back on the symptoms you had and the harmful coping strategies you used before you started working on the abuse. Help yourself become aware of any reductions in your symptoms or changes in your use of coping strategies by writing them down under the headings below. Rebecca's answers to this exercise have been written underneath each one as examples.

- **Symptoms or harmful coping strategies I no longer have:**
  I don't self injure any more.

  _____

  _____

  _____

  _____

  _____

  _____

- **Symptoms or harmful coping strategies that happen less often:**
  I occasionally have flashbacks, nightmares and hallucinations and I still isolate myself sometimes. I don't use illness as often to escape difficulties.

  _____
  _____
  _____
  _____
  _____

- **Symptoms I can cope with now:**
  I still hear negative messages in my head from those who abused me and those who should have taken care of me but I am not so afraid of them. Blanking off is less of a problem and I can stay in a situation now even if it's difficult. I still get frightened but now I am able to talk about my feelings.

  _____
  _____
  _____
  _____
  _____

- **Symptoms and harmful coping strategies I still need to work on:**
  The things I need to work on are: binge-eating, fear of sexual and non-sexual relationships and my fear of being humiliated.

  _____
  _____
  _____
  _____
  _____

Examples
Lesley-Leigh

- Symptoms or harmful coping strategies I no longer have:
  I don't take drugs and I don't drink too much now. I don't make myself sick or hurt myself anymore.
- Symptoms or harmful coping strategies that happen less often:
  I still occasionally have nightmares and flashbacks and become afraid of closing the bedroom door. I can cope with dark places more often now.

- Symptoms I can cope with now:
  I still see my abuser's face sometimes when I'm having sex but I can cope with it more easily now. I'm getting better at going to places where there are a lot of people.
- Symptoms and harmful coping strategies I still need to work on:
  I still cope at difficult times by not eating and I still look around when I'm out to see if my abusers are about. I love my kids and I need to work on showing them I love them and I really want to be able to say it to them.

Maya

- Symptoms or harmful coping strategies I no longer have:
  I don't try to 'fix' other people. I don't 'blood-let'. I don't smoke.
- Symptoms or harmful coping strategies that happen less often:
  I'm not so obsessed with exercising. I still have problems around food (binge/starve cycle), depression and 'spacing out' but they don't last as long as previously.
- Symptoms I can cope with now:
  I'm not as frightened of people's anger and I don't feel as guilty for telling about my abuse.
- Symptoms and harmful coping strategies I still need to work on:
  I still burn myself, take too many tranquillizers or drink too much alcohol when things go wrong. I am still defensive and over-controlling.

Survivor's comment

It made me realize how far I've come but I was also frightened when I saw how many symptoms I still had to work on. However, it has also made me more determined to succeed. Keep on trying – you will succeed in the end, as I will. PAULINE

EXERCISE 11.5   HOW HAVE I CHANGED? RELATIONSHIPS
Aim   To see if there are any improvements in your relationships with people and to look at what changes you still want to work on.

Think about your relationships with friends, family, sexual partners, children, work colleagues or others. Have they changed in any way? Make some notes below on any improvements in your relationships, however small, and any difficulties that still need working on. Rebecca's answers to the exercise are given as examples.

I found it easier to do the exercise by splitting it up into different categories like family, friends, work colleagues and sexual relationships and thinking about each separately. REBECCA

Positive changes in my relationships

I relate to my family on equal terms now and I have begun to relate to children. My friendships are more equal and are deeper. They are now based on mutual support not what they can give me. I also have more positive relationships at work.

_____

_____

_____

_____

_____

Relationship problems I still need to work on

I still react resentfully when my mother asks me to do things, especially when she uses manipulation and the 'poor me' trip. I need to be more assertive with people. I still need to do a lot of work on relationships that are potentially sexual.

_____

_____

_____

_____

_____

Examples
Anthony
Positive changes in my relationships:

I can talk openly to the family about the abuse and don't fly off the handle when the abuser's name is mentioned. I know now that I have some very good friends who know I have been abused and will listen to me when I get down in the dumps.

Relationship problems I still need to work on:

I still get angry with people and I have to work on my temper which I lose at times. Sometimes when I'm out with my mates I find it difficult to be with people and I just take off. I know they worry about me. It's when I'm on my own like that when self-harm might happen.

Pauline

Positive changes in my relationships:

> I can now feel more equal with my partner. I do not take my feelings out on my child.

Relationship problems I still need to work on:

> I still give in to what other people want.

Survivor's comment

> This exercise made me happy because it helped me see that there *are* positive developments in my present relationships. It also gave me a focus for other areas to improve. REBECCA

The betrayal involved in sexual abuse often results in problems in some or all of the Survivor's later relationships. Be aware of any small improvements you have made in your relationships and remember you can continue working on making your relationships better. After doing the exercises in this book you may feel better about yourself and have worked through your feelings about other people. Making these changes in yourself can help you in your relationships with others but sometimes it is necessary to work with a therapist to improve your relationships. If you still have serious problems in your relationships you may want to think about seeking individual or group therapy.

The first four exercises aimed to help you see any progress you have made in the way you think and feel, in your symptoms and ways of coping, and in your relationships:

> Looking back at the way my life was I can see the progress I've made now. CATHERINE

There will almost certainly be areas you still need to work on – self-development is a lifelong task. For now try to focus on the positive changes you have made; later in the chapter we will be looking at the things you still need to work on.

My progress

> Looking at the ways I have improved made me feel excited and gave me a sense of achievement. REBECCA

The next exercise helps you pull together the changes you have made in different parts of your life and celebrate any progress you have made so far. Representing your journey to healing in some way can help you see where you have come from, where you are now, and increase your awareness of the changes you have made.

Children have to use all the resources available to them to find ways of living through the trauma of sexual abuse and keeping some part of themselves safe. Finding ways of surviving sexual abuse is a creative process. Many Survivors produce imaginative writing, poetry and artwork. You may enjoy using your creativity to represent your journey towards healing and to celebrate your progress.

EXERCISE 11.6   MY PROGRESS

Aim   To represent and celebrate your journey towards breaking free from the effects of the abuse.

Represent the changes you have made so far in one of the ways suggested below. This exercise is *not* about what you still have to do but is a way of focusing on the positive steps you have already made and celebrating your courage and success. Choose the way that suits you and enjoy yourself.

- Draw or paint yourself and your life at the beginning of your journey to healing and where you are now.

  Or

- Draw a cartoon strip showing the stages you have been through.

  Or

- Represent your journey through poetry, music or dance.

  Or

- Write about any positive changes you are aware of in yourself or your life since you started working on the abuse. You could write about how you overcame any difficulties you faced and about any changes in the way you feel about yourself. What are the things you now enjoy about yourself and your life?

My progress

Examples
Maya

Striding out
Purposefully,
Strong and upright
Along the path of freedom.
Treading softly,
Tentatively,
Feeling my way forwards.
Leaping, sprinting,
Scaling great heights.
Trudging wearily,
Stumbling, falling,
Finding a shoulder
To lean on
Until refreshed.
I start again,
Unfettered.
Experiencing life anew.
Reborn
After therapy.

Pauline
Pauline created this way of representing the stages she has moved through:

I chose a load of different outfits from my wardrobe and I taped some songs. I started off by sitting in the corner crying like a lost orphan and I played *Amazing Grace*. I continued by changing my clothes and changing my image as I played different songs. As I went along I felt stronger and more positive until I ended up wearing a red dress with my hair piled up, with high heeled shoes on and a red handbag. I felt ever so powerful and I played *Simply the Best*.

I felt very emotional expressing the stages I have gone through, right up to when I felt very strong and powerful. It really helped me get things out of my system. Everyone has to find the way that suits them but this worked wonders for me!

Maintaining progress and dealing with relapses

Becoming aware of the changes I have made initially made me scared that although I have moved on a lot things could still go pear-shaped. REBECCA

Looking at your progress may give you a sense of achievement but it can also make you afraid of slipping back to how you were. At certain times you may find it difficult to cope. It is a normal part of life to have good and bad days. You may become distressed by situations that remind you of your abuse or you may be suffering from the normal stresses of life. At these times distressing feelings from the past can return and you may revert to old harmful ways of coping. This can make you think you have gone back to square one instead of understanding that you are having a temporary setback. The next exercise asks you to produce a list of non-harmful coping strategies for use during difficult times.

EXERCISE 11.7   POSITIVE COPING STRATEGIES I USE NOW
Aim   To have a list of non-harmful coping strategies ready to use when you are feeling bad.

By now you may have replaced some of your harmful coping strategies with more of the non-harmful ones. Write a list here of the positive ways you now use to cope when you are under stress or feeling bad.

Positive coping strategies

_____

_____

_____

_____

_____

_____

_____

_____

_____

_____

_____

Examples
Lesley-Leigh

Keep my mind busy.
Get out of the house.
Talk to others.
Go for a walk or a drive.
Clean a cupboard out.
Do something positive.
Have a good cry.
Deal with my problems a bit at a time.

Rebecca

Now when I'm having difficulties I:
Ask for help.
Write things down.
Challenge negative self talk.
Seek out friends instead of spending all my time alone.
Draw my feelings.
Do a sculpt of my feelings.
Write down/draw or sculpt nightmares and hallucinations.
Get out and about instead of giving in to depression.
Work through them rather than let them destroy me.

Anthony

Writing letters to my abuser (not to send) to express my feelings.
Helping people and listening to other people's problems helps me realize I am
   not alone.
Keeping busy.
If I'm feeling really bad I'll phone the Samaritans.
Talking to my close friends.

Pauline

I challenge my negative thinking and try to remember everything I've learnt. I try to put it into practice. Sometimes it helps to sit and cry.

Maya

If I have a bad day I do not panic as much now and I tell myself everyone has bad days at times. Instead of avoiding my problems I am more likely to face them by writing them down, expressing my feelings and taking some action rather than giving in and feeling helpless. This helps me control my mood swings. I don't get as high these days and my lows don't last as long. My dog is a very positive influence on me. I hug her, kiss her, stroke her, cry on her and she doesn't mind at all. She needs a lot of exercise so I have something to get out of bed for and the walks do me good.

Your positive coping strategies may help you overcome your difficulties, but sometimes you may continue to feel bad or have symptoms return for a longer period. The next exercise suggests some ways of dealing with relapses. It is much more difficult to think of positive things when you are feeling bad so spend some time now, or when you are in a positive mood, thinking of what you can do to help yourself if you do go through a difficult phase.

It is important that you do this exercise when you are feeling positive so all your helpful suggestions are ready for you when you feel down. REBECCA

EXERCISE 11.8   POSITIVE WAYS OF DEALING WITH RELAPSES
Aim   To look at ways of dealing with relapses and continuing the progress you have made.

Read through the list below of positive ways of dealing with relapses and add any others you can think of.

Positive ways of dealing with relapses
Tell myself it's normal to have relapses occasionally and that I can get through it.
Remember I've felt this bad before and it will pass.
Take one day at a time.
Remind myself of the progress I have made and that this is a temporary setback – I am *not* back at square one.
Write down how I'm feeling.
Try to use my positive coping strategies – see list in Exercise 11.7 above.
Go through Chapters 3 and 4 on coping strategies and dealing with symptoms again.
Talk to a friend.
Contact one of the people on my list from Exercise 1.1.
Work through this book again.
Contact my GP.
Phone the Samaritans or another telephone help-line.
Get some professional support or therapy.
Think about how far I've come and how I'm going to persevere with the journey.

_____
_____
_____
_____
_____
_____
_____
_____
_____
_____

Remember you are not alone, asking for help is a positive coping strategy.

Example

I think of the positive changes that have happened.
I pray.
I say self-affirmations like 'you are doing well'.
I contact friends.
I treat myself.
CALLI

Survivors' comments

I can't deny that some weeks I can feel quite down and may even feel like I'm slipping back but then I remember how far I've come and I soon turn things around. I decided my abuser wasn't going to win. With that thought in mind I can wade through the bad stuff. ANITA B

I coped with my fear of it all going wrong by writing down all my positive coping strategies and remembering all the useful contacts and support I have now. I also know that I've pulled myself up before so I can do it again. REBECCA

It helps to know it's natural to have a relapse so you don't feel a failure when it happens. I did have a relapse and I was terrified and thought everything was happening all over again and I'd never get out of it. I got some help and now I'm loads better again. PAULINE

If you begin to feel distressed or down remember to turn to these exercises and remind yourself of the non-harmful coping strategies you can use and the things that can help you cope with relapses.

What I still want to do

It may now be a good time to think about what you still want to do and what kind of a person you would like to be when you have overcome the constraints of your past. You will probably still need to work on issues and problems resulting from the abuse and still want to make changes in yourself and your life. When you were a child the adults around you may have had expectations of how they wanted you to be or told you how you were going to turn out but now try to think about how *you* would like to be in the future.

EXERCISE 11.9   WHAT I STILL WANT TO DO
Aim   To look at what you still want to achieve on your journey towards breaking free of the past.

Spend some time thinking about any changes you still want to make in:
The way you live.
Your interests/hobbies.

Your job/occupation/career.
Qualifications or skills.
The way you look.
Your marriage, partnership, sexual relationships or love-life.
Your friendships or other relationships.
The kind of person you are (personality, strengths, attributes, personal style).

Also think about:
What you still want to do.
The problems you still need to solve.

What I still want to do.
Here are some suggestions of ways to represent what you still want to do and how you would like to be in the future. Try all of them or choose the one that suits you.

- Write a description of your future self using the list above to help you. You may find it easier to write in the third person rather than using 'I'. For example: 'Amanda is a strong person. She is very kind to other people but she also knows how to look after herself.'
- Do a drawing or a cartoon strip of the life you would like to lead and how you would like to be.
- Fill in the shapes on the next page.

Use this space to write a description of the person you would like to be or do a drawing.

What I still want to do

Fill in the shapes with the things you still want to change in your life. (See example below.)

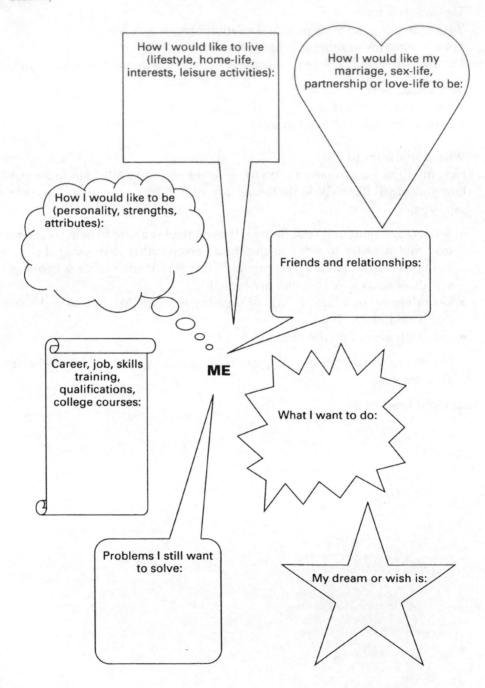

How I would like to live (lifestyle, home-life, interests, leisure activities):

How I would like my marriage, sex-life, partnership or love-life to be:

How I would like to be (personality, strengths, attributes):

Friends and relationships:

Career, job, skills training, qualifications, college courses:

ME

What I want to do:

Problems I still want to solve:

My dream or wish is:

Example

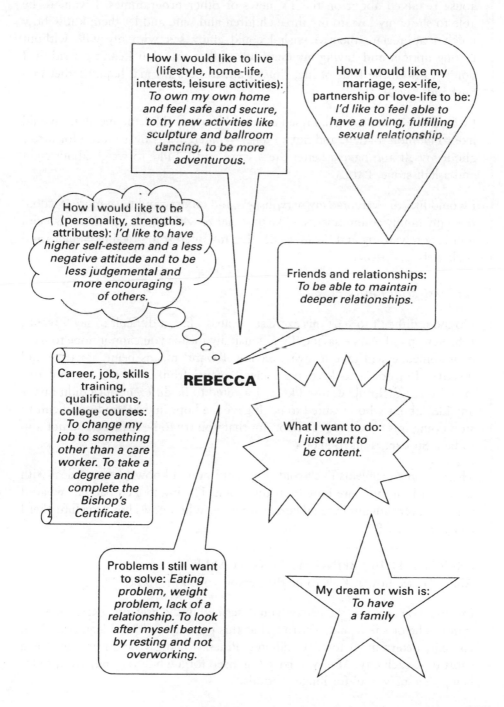

How I would like to live
(lifestyle, home-life,
interests, leisure activities):
*To own my own home
and feel safe and secure,
to try new activities like
sculpture and ballroom
dancing, to be more
adventurous.*

How I would like my
marriage, sex-life,
partnership or love-life to be:
*I'd like to feel able to
have a loving, fulfilling
sexual relationship.*

How I would like to be
(personality, strengths,
attributes): *I'd like to have
higher self-esteem and a less
negative attitude and to be
less judgemental and
more encouraging
of others.*

Friends and relationships:
*To be able to maintain
deeper relationships.*

REBECCA

Career, job, skills
training,
qualifications,
college courses:
*To change my
job to something
other than a care
worker. To take a
degree and
complete the
Bishop's
Certificate.*

What I want to do:
*I just want to
be content.*

Problems I still want
to solve: *Eating
problem, weight
problem, lack of a
relationship. To look
after myself better
by resting and not
overworking.*

My dream or wish is:
*To have
a family*

I would like to be able to get on with my life without getting angry whenever abuse is talked about on the TV news or other programmes. I want to be able to show my love to my three children and wife and let them know how much I appreciate them. I wish I could enjoy sex with my wife without getting uptight and having my mind full of thoughts that I can't get rid of. I don't want all the frills of life, I just want to be a normal happy father and husband. GRAHAM

I would like to be strong in myself and be able to say 'No' and mean it. I would like to be more patient and not so quick-tempered. I want to feel a lot better about myself and have a better dress sense and I'd like to weigh about eight and a half stone. PAULA

I would like to overcome my nervousness and anxiety and have more freedom from my family commitments. I like to socialize with my caring friends which I find very rewarding and I want to develop my interest in breeding budgies and cockatiels. ANTHONY

Survivors' comments

I found it difficult to start this exercise because I find it difficult to say 'I want'. It brings up old fears – saying 'I want' usually means you cannot hope to have it or someone will take it away. Saying 'I want' means being assertive and positive. I'm going to keep on using 'I want' from now on. I found this exercise very helpful because I knew I wanted to be different but I didn't have any idea about who I wanted to be. It gave me hope and I found it difficult to stop doing this exercise! It's important that you try to be realistic and not aim to be a Superperson. REBECCA

There's some problems I've avoided up until now. I know I have to deal with them but I am not sure how to at this point. Having looked back to where I was – I never thought I would be as I am now. Who knows how much further I can go? ANITA B

EXERCISE 11.10   BEING MY FUTURE SELF
Aim   To see how it feels to be the person you want to be.

Imagine you are now the person you described in the previous exercise. Sit or stand as he or she would. Try to feel as this person would feel (e.g. confident, content, determined) for five minutes. Practise being your future self for a short time each day. After you have practised for a while you may want to try being this 'new you' for longer periods.

Survivors' comments

I have tried being this kind of person and I do feel a lot better about myself. When I try to be my ideal self I always sit up straight. I seem to laugh more and feel more confident. PAULA

A good self-reflective exercise whether you have been abused or not. A positive approach to the future, making me feel more self-confident and in control if I take the chance. CATHERINE

EXERCISE 11.11   MAKING CHANGES

Aim   To help you plan the changes you want to make in your life.

1   Look back over Exercise 11.9 and think of two or three things you would like to change about yourself or your life. Choose the easiest ones first. It is important that you choose small changes that you are able to do now. For example:

- changing your hairstyle
- asking people to call you Amanda instead of Mandy
- joining an assertion course
- taking exercise
- applying for a course
- buying clothes to suit the 'new' you
- trying to feel better about yourself by continuing working through this book or doing something for yourself every day.

Write them here.

I would like to:
(E.g. I would like to learn to cook better.)

-
-
-

2   Think of ways of achieving each one. Write down how you will do it.

I will do it by:
(E.g. I could sign up for an evening class.)

-
-
-

3 What is stopping you making these changes?
  (*E.g. I'm scared of going to the adult learning centre.*)

  -
  -
  -

4 How can you overcome these obstacles?
  (*E.g. I could ask a friend to go with me.*)

  -
  -
  -

Why not start now? If you can't start straight away set yourself a date when you will begin to make these changes in your life.

When you have achieved these changes you may want to think of three more small steps.

Examples
Paula
I would like to:

- Lose weight.
- Control my temper.
- Change my dress sense.

I will do it by:

- I am on a diet to lose weight.
- I sit in a room on my own to control my temper.
- I have started to buy and wear bright coloured clothes.

Anita B
I would like to:

- Become more assertive.
- Gain more qualifications.
- Believe in myself.

I will do it by:

- Taking an assertion course.
- Enrolling at college.
- Hopefully by doing both of the above I will learn to believe in myself.

Survivors' comments

> I found these exercises very helpful and think it is useful to return to them at different stages of the healing process. I needed to focus on what was stopping me becoming the person I wanted to be. I realized that I unconsciously needed to be a victim (as an adult) because I was too scared to be anything else – it was all I'd ever known. SARAH

> I've never dared look at what the future may hold before. ANITA B

> Doing the exercises in this chapter made me realize how much the abuse has affected me. It was very hard to look deep into my self and I had a lot of mixed feelings about where I am now and where I would like to be. It was also difficult to realize I have to make changes in myself in order to feel happy. By doing these exercises you *can* begin to make changes in your life. LESLEY-LEIGH

In the past your life and your feelings were controlled by other people. Thinking of a positive future for yourself and taking even tiny steps towards it can make you feel more in control of your own life. Keep returning to these exercises and plan a few more small steps forward. Step by step you can walk towards the life you want to have even though it may be a long and difficult journey. Try to see there is a light at the end of the tunnel and head towards it.

The next step

The aim of this book is to help you begin the process of working through your problems and accepting yourself more so you can move on through your life without the shadow of the past. The important thing is that you have started the process, not whether you have made big or small steps forward. Try not to compare your progress with that of the Survivors who have contributed examples and quotations to this book.

Some of you will feel you have worked on your abuse enough, at least for now, and have achieved as much as you want to at this point. You may understand more about what happened to you and who was really responsible for the abuse. You may now want to put the abuse behind you and continue creating your own future. Some of you may wish to join awareness or support groups for Survivors. Some Survivors join campaigning groups, but remember it is important to sort out your own feelings and problems before you try to help other people.

> Doing these exercises has brought a lot of things up for me. I am feeling very mixed up at the moment. I feel I have come on a lot but I still have a long way to go. Before I was in a tunnel with no light, now I'm beginning to see a little light. I have to come to terms with a lot of things which, before doing these

exercises, I could put to the back of my mind. I feel I want some therapy again because there are things I want to talk about and I want to deal with for my own sake as well as my family's. LESLEY-LEIGH

Like Lesley-Leigh many of you will have found that working through this book has stirred up thoughts and feelings that you still need to work on. You may want to do this by continuing to work on the exercises in this book or continuing with therapy you are currently involved with. You may feel you are now ready to go for some individual or group therapy; asking for therapy may be difficult but it can also be the way to receive the help you deserve. The Sources of Help section at the back of the book suggests ways of finding a therapist.

I was very frightened at the idea of therapy. It was the thought of other people knowing I was abused. I was also scared of not being believed. I told someone and I was believed and that was my first step forward. Now I am not bothered who knows that I have been abused. I am not ashamed, I didn't do anything wrong. LESLEY-LEIGH

The last exercise asks you to give yourself some time to think about what *you* want to do next. It is not about what you *should* do but about what is the right thing for you.

EXERCISE 11.12   THE NEXT STEP?
Aim   To help you think about what you are going to do now.

Now you have nearly finished this book it is time to think about what you want to do next. Read the following list and tick off any of the things that seem right for you.

What do you want to do now?	Applies to you?
Take a well-earned break	_____
Take a break then continue working on my problems	_____
Get some therapy or professional help	_____
Continue with my therapy	_____
Join a Survivors' group	_____
Carry on working through this book	_____
Go on an assertion or confidence-building course	_____
Get on with my life	_____
Carry on developing my potential	_____
Meet or network with other Survivors	_____
Campaign for awareness of childhood abuse and for resources for Survivors	_____
Celebrate my progress	_____

Write down anything else you would like to do now:

_____
_____
_____
_____
_____
_____
_____
_____

Write down the steps you can take to achieve this:

_____
_____
_____
_____
_____
_____
_____
_____

Examples

Pauline

I want to:

> Take a well-earned break.
> Get on with my life and put the abuse behind me.
> Carry on developing my potential.
> Network with other Survivors.

I will do this by:

> Doing a course in interior design.
> Attending a local support group for Survivors.

Maya

I want to:

> Relax – chill out and take life as it comes.

I will do this by:

> Having fun, riding my bike, painting, playing with the dog, jumping in puddles, flying a kite, taking some kids out. Sitting in the garden on my lounger and

lounging. Having some aromatherapy. Going to the pub and having a laugh with friends. Having sex in the shower (with my husband)!

Calli

I want to:

> Take another holiday.
> Make some new friends.
> Write a book.
> Realize the wealth of potential within.
> Live life to the full.

I will do this by:

> Taking all opportunities as they arise.

Survivor's comment

> This exercise made me feel some fear about the future. It really helped me to acknowledge my feelings of fear about the future and also my fear of letting go of the past and moving on. REBECCA

It takes a lot of courage to read this book, look back on a painful part of your life and work through the distressing feelings and problems that often result from childhood abuse. We hope you have made some progress in breaking free from your past and that you now have hopes for the future. Society still has a long way to go towards providing help for child and adult Survivors, providing treatment for abusers and changing the legal system to be more responsive to child abuse. Society is, however, at last facing up to the reality and scale of child abuse. Perhaps we can celebrate the progress we have made as a society and as individuals in recognizing child abuse and acknowledging and helping its victims.

> Keep on moving on! REBECCA

How I feel now

It seems fitting to end this book with some words of encouragement from Survivors. Some of them are at the beginning of their journey while others are receiving or have completed individual or group therapy as well as completing the exercises in this book. We asked them to write about 'how I feel now'.

Anita B was raped by a family friend, starting when she was 8 years old.

> The exercises made me think about things which I would have preferred to leave alone. At the time it caused all sorts of emotions to be stirred up and I

felt worse than when I started. But I stuck with it and it did get better. Actually seeing your thoughts and feelings on paper seemed to put things in perspective. I feel much better now than I did. My confidence and self-esteem are higher than I've ever known. My life is entirely different now. I see things clearly and I stand up for myself (something I've never done). Before if anything went wrong I would think it was my fault but not anymore. I feel like I'm a 'real' person now, not just a front for others to see.

Pauline was sexually, physically and emotionally abused by many individuals both inside and outside her family.

I was too shy and scared to go for therapy in case they thought I was mad and locked me up. I did it, I got up the courage and went. I now feel great, most of the time I can be myself and be what I've always wanted to be.

Danny was physically and emotionally abused in his childhood by his parents and while in care.

I feel stronger in myself. I feel on the road to recovery. I also feel it is possible to combine the two extreme sides of my self to make a more interesting whole. I'm more positive, less aggressive and use my brain more. It's too early yet to say where it will lead to. It's getting better by degrees but it can require a lot of mental effort. On a good day I feel optimistic about the future because I like myself more than I used to. There are more good days now. It's still hard to fight back from a bad day but the less booze I drink the easier it is.

Jean was sexually abused by her father.

I'm beginning to accept that the abuse was not my fault and that I could not have prevented what happened. I am now releasing all the pent-up emotions I kept at bay for most of my life: the guilt of blaming myself, feeling dirty. It's helped to find out that I'm not going insane because I was talking to people that only I could see. I'm beginning to see that there could be a light at the end of the tunnel after all. I'm determined to finally free myself of my abuser.

Catherine was sexually abused by her father.

Before I didn't know if I belonged in my mind or body. Now I feel free, light and optimistic but, most importantly, I feel like me. Going through a bad life experience has made me into a good person. Now I feel equal to most people. I like myself. I enjoy friendships. I see lots ahead.

Graham was sexually abused by his mother and her friends.

I am not near the end of my therapy yet but I think it's working. I feel a lot better having someone to talk to. I do have off days but I think I'm coping and getting on.

Sarah was neglected and physically abused by her family and was also sexually abused both within and outside her family. She finished therapy some time ago and is now a counsellor herself.

> I am stronger and in touch with reality now. I understand myself and my emotions much more. When I look back to who I was and who I have become I feel proud. It's been hard work but worthwhile. I do believe I could survive almost anything now. I feel so different. I wouldn't say I was fully healed because that would mean I was perfect and I want to continue exploring my *self*. It is strange sometimes when I hear my own clients and remember I once felt like they do. I feel good knowing how far I have come. No longer a victim or a Survivor, I'm me.

Calli was abused by an organized group of people including her own family.

> I feel a sense of achievement. I no longer want to look back on my abuse. I prefer to look forward to the changes within that are enabling me to function as a 'human being'. I believe I can live and enjoy life – I have confidence in me.

We admire your courage and wish you well.

Further Reading

Self-help books for Survivors

Ainscough, Carolyn and Toon, Kay, *Breaking Free: Help for Survivors of Child Sexual Abuse*. Sheldon Press, 1993, new edition 2000.

Davis, Laura, *The Courage to Heal: A Guide for Women Survivors of Child Sexual Abuse*. Bass, Ellen and Cedar, 1990.

Gil, Eliana, *Outgrowing the Pain: A Book for and about Adults Abused as Children*. Rockville, MD: Launch, 1983.

Parkes, Penny, *Rescuing the Inner Child: Therapy for Adults Sexually Abused as Children*. Souvenir Press (E & A) Ltd, 1989.

Sanford, Linda T., *Strong at the Broken Places: Overcoming the Trauma of Childhood Abuse*. Virago, 1990.

Mines, Stephanie, *Sexual Abuse, Sacred Wound – Transforming Deep Trauma*. Station Hill Openings, 1996. The role of expressive and creative work in healing from sexual abuse.

Wood, Wendy and Hatton, Lesley, *Triumph over Darkness: Understanding and Healing the Trauma of Childhood Sexual Abuse*. Beyond Words Publishing Inc., 1988.

For Survivors abused by women

Elliott, Michele, (ed), *Female Sexual Abuse of Children: The Ultimate Taboo*. Longman, 1993.

For black women Survivors

Wilson, Melba, *Crossing the Boundary: Black Women Survive Incest*. Virago, 1993.

For male Survivors

Etherington, Kim, *Adult Male Survivors of Sexual Abuse*. Pitman Publishing, 1995.

Grubman-Black, S. D., *Broken Boys/Mending Men: Recovery from Childhood Sexual Abuse*. Blue Ridge Summit, PA: Tab Books, 1990.

Hunter, Mic, *Abused Boys: The Neglected Victims of Sexual Abuse*. MA:Lexington, 1990.

Lew, Mike, *Victims no longer: Men recovering from Incest and other Sexual Child Abuse*. New York Neuraumont Publishers, 1988.

For Survivors with learning disabilities

Hollins, Sheila, and Sinason, Valerie, *Bob Tells All*. St George's Hospital Mental Health Library, 1992.

Hollins, Sheila, and Sinason, Valerie, *Jenny Speaks Out*. St George's Hospital Mental Health Library, 1992.

Writings by Survivors

Farthing, Linda, Malone, Caroline, Marce, Lorraine, (eds), *The Memory Bird: Survivors of Sexual Abuse*. Virago, 1996. More than 200 male and female contributors.

Autobiography

Angelou, Maya, *I Know Why the Caged Bird Sings*. Virago, 1983.

Chase, Trudi, *When Rabbit Howls*. Sidgwick and Jackson 1998. The story of a woman who developed multiple personalities to survive her abuse.

Fraser, Sylvia, *My Father's House – A Memoir of Incest and of Healing*. Virago, 1989.

Spring, Jacqueline, *Cry Hard and Swim*. Virago, 1987.

Fiction

Walker, Alice, *The Colour Purple*. London: Women's Press, 1983.

For partners and families of Survivors

Davis, Laura, *Allies in Healing: When the Person you Love was Sexually Abused as a Child*. New York: Harper Perennial, 1991.

Graber, Ken, *Ghosts in the Bedroom: A Guide for Partners of Incest Survivors*. Health Communication, 1988.

Messages from Parents whose Children have been Sexually Abused. The Child and Family Resource Group, Leeds Community and Mental Health Trust, Belmont House, 3/5 Belmont Grove, Leeds LS2 9NP.

From Discovery to Recovery: A Parent's Survival Guide to Child Sexual Abuse.
Warwickshire Social Services department, PO Box 48, Shire Hall, Warwick
CV34 4RD. Audio tape and booklet.

Help with relationships

Litvinoff, Sarah, *The Relate Guide to Better Relationships.* Ebury Press, 1991.
Secunda, Victoria, *When you and your Mother can't be Friends.* Cedar, 1992.

For therapists

Hall, Liz, and Lloyd, Siobhan, *Surviving Child Sexual Abuse: A Handbook for
Helping Women Challenge their Past.* Lewes: Falmer Press, 1989.

Books referred to in the text

Finkelhor, D., *Child Sexual Abuse: New Theory and Research.* New York: Free
Press, 1984.
Finkelhor, D., *A Sourcebook in Child Sexual Abuse.* Sage, 1986.

Note: There are more books listed in *Breaking Free* which may help you
manage your symptoms, work on your relationships and protect your
children from abuse.

Sources of Help

A GP, health visitor, social worker or other professional can assist you in getting help from a clinical psychologist or other therapist. Do not be afraid to ask to see a woman if you feel uncomfortable talking to a man (or vice versa).

The national addresses or phone numbers for various organizations are listed below. For information on local sources of help contact the national office or try your local Telephone Directory. Please include a stamped self-addressed envelope for written replies.

Telephone helplines

The organizations listed below offer someone to talk to, advice and sometimes face-to-face counselling.

ChildLine

Children can phone **0800 1111** (free) or write to Freepost NATN1111, London, E1 6BR, if they are in trouble or are being abused.

NCH

For children and adults.
08457 626579

NSPCC

For parents, children, abusers and professionals.
0808 800 500 (24-hour helpline)

Rape and Sexual Abuse Support Centre

Monday–Friday 12.00–12.30 pm and 7.00 pm–9.30 pm.
Weekends and Bank Holidays 2.30 pm–5.00 pm.
08451 221331

SAFE: Supporting Survivors of Satanic Abuse

Helpline for survivors of ritual and satanic abuse. Offers counselling, listening, advice and referrals.
Wednesday 6.30 pm–8.30 pm, Thursday 7.00 pm–9.00 pm.
PO Box 1557, Salisbury, SP1 2TP.
01722 410889

Samaritans

24-hour listening and befriending service for the lonely, suicidal or depressed. Find the number of your local group in the phone book.

Preventing abuse

Phone one of the helplines listed above or contact the following agencies if you suspect a child is being abused or is at risk of abuse, or you know of an abuser who has any contact with children.

Police

Many districts now have a special Police Unit that works with sexual abuse. Phone your local police station and ask to speak to the officer who deals with sexual abuse.

Social Services

Phone your local office and ask for the Child Protection Officer or the Duty Officer.

If you are abusing children or have urges to abuse children phone the NSPCC or contact Social Services or the Police.

Therapy/counselling and support

British Association for Counselling and Psychotherapy

BACP House, 15 St John's Business Park, Lutterworth, LE17 4HB.
0870 443 5252
01455 883300
Email: bacp@bacp.co.uk
Website: http://www.bacp.co.uk

Children 1st

83 Whitehouse Loan, Edinburgh, EH9 1AT.
Headquarters: **0131 446 2300**
ParentLine Scotland: **0808 800 2222**
Website: http://www.children1st.org.uk

Citizens' Advice Bureau

Can direct you to local groups who can help. Find the number of your nearest office in the phone book.

Clinical psychologists

Your GP can refer you to a clinical psychologist or you can ask another professional for advice on how to get to see a psychologist.

DABS (Directory & Book Services)

DABS collate information and produce a national directory for resources for survivors. They also provide an excellent mail order service for books.
4 New Hill, Conisbrough, Doncaster, DN12 3HA.
01709 860023 (telephone and fax)
Website: http://www.dabsbooks.co.uk

MIND

Offers individual counselling and group work.
Information Helpline: Monday–Friday 9.15 am–5.15 pm.
0845 7660163
Email: info@mind.org.uk
Website: http://www.mind.org.uk

NCH

Provides national network of child sexual abuse treatment centres – providing support and counselling for children and their families. Adult survivors also.
85 Highbury Park, London, N5 1UD.
020 7704 7000
Website: http://www.nch.org.uk

Rape and Sexual Abuse Support Centre

PO Box 383, Croydon, Surrey, CR9 2AW.
020 8683 3311

RELATE

Can help with relationship difficulties and sexual problems. Provides couple counselling.
Premier House, Carolina Court, Lakeside, Doncaster, South Yorkshire, DN4 5RA.
0845 456 1310
Email: enquiries@relate.org.uk
Website: http://www.relate.org.uk

Victim Support

Co-ordinates nation-wide victim support schemes. Trained volunteers offer practical and emotional help to the victims of crime including rape and sexual assault.
Cranmer House, 39 Brixton Road, London, SW9 6DZ.
020 7735 9166

Women's Therapy Centre

Offers group and individual therapy.
10 Manor Gardens, London, N7 6JS.
Psychotherapy enquiries:
020 7263 6200 (Tuesday and Wednesday 2.00 pm–4.00 pm and Thursday 12.00–2.00 pm)
appointments@womenstherapycentre.co.uk
General enquiries: **020 7263 7860**
Email: info@womenstherapycentre.co.uk
Website: http://www.womenstherapycentre.co.uk

Special agencies

ACT (Ann Craft Trust)

Provides an information and networking service to adult and child survivors with learning disabilities and workers involved in this area.
Monday–Thursday 8.30 am–5.00 pm, Friday 8.30 am–2 pm.
Centre for Social Work, University Park, Nottingham, NG7 2RD.
0115 951 5400
Email: ann-craft-trust@nottingham.ac.uk
Website: http://www.anncrafttrust.org

Accuracy About Abuse

Information service. Background to media controversies.
Website: http://www.accuracyaboutabuse.org

Beacon Foundation

Services for survivors of satanic/ritualistic abuse and their carers and support for professionals.
Weekdays 10.00 am–4.00 pm.
3 Grosvenor Avenue, Rhyl, Clwyd, LL18 4HA.
01745 343600 (helpline)
Website: http://www.napac.org.uk/survivors/support/groups/detail.asp?id=546

Kidscape

Information on protecting children.
020 7730 3300

London Lesbian and Gay Switchboard

020 7837 7324
Website: http://www.llgs.org.uk

National Association of Christian Survivors of Sexual Abuse

An interdenominational organization run by survivors for survivors.
C/o 38 Sydenham Villas Road, Cheltenham, Glos., GL52 6DZ.
Website: http://www.napac.org.uk/survivors/support/groups/detail.asp?id=501

NAPAC (National Association of People Abused in Childhood)

Organizes an annual march through London in the autumn for survivors and their supporters and is setting up a national database of support for survivors.
42 Curtain Road, London, EC2A 3NH.
0800 085 3330 (support line)

National Deaf Children's Society

Agency catering for deaf children and their families. Can offer books/info to professionals.
15 Dufferin Street, London, EC1Y 8UR.
020 7490 8656
Email: ndcs@ndcs.org.uk
Website: http://www.ndcs.org.uk

RAINS (Ritualised Abuse: Information and Support Group)

Professional network to help those who are supporting survivors of ritual abuse.
Jeff Hopkins, Lecturer in Social Work, Department of Applied Social Studies, Keele University, Keele, ST5 5BG.

Index

NOTES

NOTES

NOTES

NOTES

NOTES

NOTES